CARING
FOR YOUR
AGING PARENTS

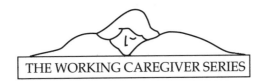

THE WORKING CAREGIVER SERIES

CARING

FOR YOUR

AGING PARENTS

*A Sourcebook of
Timesaving Techniques and Tips*

· · · · · · · · ·

Kerri S. Smith

ADVISORY PANEL
Susan C. Aldridge, Ph.D.
Susan Fox Buchanan
Pamela A. Erickson, R.N.
Virginia Fraser
Milton Hanson, LCSW
Susan Hellman
Lewis Kallas
Maria Kallas
Mary Kouri, Ph.D.
Crispin Sargent
Edith Sherman, Ph.D.
John Torres

 AMERICAN SOURCE BOOKS

Lakewood • Colorado

This book is dedicated to my heroes and role models, Bonnie and Charles Smith.

Book design and series logo by Karen Groves
Cover design by Elaine Duncan

ATTENTION ORGANIZATIONS AND CORPORATIONS:
This book is available at quantity discounts on bulk purchases for educational, business, or sales promotional use. For further information, please contact American Source Books, PO Box 280353, Lakewood, CO 80228, (303) 980-0580.

Library of Congress Cataloging-in Publication Data

Smith, Kerri S., 1960-
      Caring for your aging parents: a sourcebook of timesaving
  techniques and tips / Kerri S. Smith.
          p.   cm.—(The Working caregiver series)
      Includes index.
      ISBN 0-9621333-8-8 (paper) :
      1. Aging parents—Care—United States. 2. Aging parents—Health
  and hygiene—United States. 3. Aged—Services for—United States.
  4. Adult children—United States. 5. Caregivers—United States.
  I. Title. II. Series.
  HV1461.S555 1992
  362.6'0973—dc20   91-33909

Printed and bound in the United States of America

9 8 7 6 5 4 3 2 1

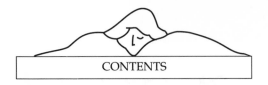

CONTENTS

CHAPTER ONE
THE HEALTH SNAPSHOT 15
. . . .

What's really wrong with your parent? How to find out everything you need to know about his or her health—learn how to pick up on symptoms and compensate for functional problems—work with your parent's doctors to coordinate whole-person health care—set up a caregiving directory of professionals to help you by telephone.

CHAPTER TWO
MODIFYING THE HOME ENVIRONMENT 23
. . . .

A step-by-step guide to making your parent's home safer and more convenient. Over 100 simple tips on rearranging the bedroom, bathroom, living room, kitchen and yard—remodeling plans—types of useful medical equipment and gadgets—where to buy what you need—ideas on do-it-yourself caregiving aids.

CHAPTER THREE
WHERE TO GET HELP 33
. . . .

Everything on accessing the elder care network in your community. You'll learn how to find free or low-cost government assistance programs—how to select and hire paid caregivers and services—which companies offer discounts and special services to seniors—how to put it all together and custom-craft your caregiving network.

How working caregivers can stay sane, healthy and happy. Practical suggestions on combining family and caregiving time—simple stress management techniques—how and when to ask for help—reclaiming your life.

ACKNOWLEDGMENTS

. . . .

To my sister and best friend Lee Wineteer, and to Rodney, the quiet genius, my appreciation for our California getaways. Those weekends kept me sane and creative while deadlines loomed.

To my brother Clifford, and Marianne, whose good-humored technical assistance made this project possible, a huge thank you and a promise—no more long-distance computer trouble-shooting calls. To Sean and Kelly, thank you for making me so happy.

For sharing her knowledge and experiences as a geriatric nurse, I thank the wonderful wild-woman, Julie Knapp Driscoll. My appreciation also to Rose Beetem, a friend and editor who helped research this book, and to Mary Throne, for her sound legal advise and 15 years of friendship.

To the hundreds of elder care professionals who graciously contributed their time and insight, my sincere thanks. And to the working caregivers whose words light up this book—Peggy, Dorothy, Joyce, Barbara, Antonia, Kim, Shirley, Caroline and Helen—thank you for sharing your lives.

I'd also like to thank the twelve panel members who reviewed the book and whipped it into shape: Susan C. Aldridge, Susan Fox Buchanan, Pamela Erickson, Virginia Fraser, Milton Hanson, Susan Hellman, Maria Kallas, Lewis Kallas, Mary Kouri, Crispin Sargent, Edith Sherman and John Torres. And to my publisher Steve Phillips, whose patience and professional expertise made things so easy, a very big thank you.

Finally, I'd like to thank Dorotha Main Harman, my tree-climbing grandma who told me to pursue my dreams.

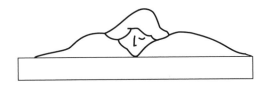

INTRODUCTION

· · · · · · · · ·

MOST WORKING CAREGIVERS LABOR UNDER THE DIFFICULT BURDEN of too much work, stress and responsibility. Family life, money and free time are taken over by another's needs.

As a working caregiver, you are well aware of the problems. What you need are quick, effective solutions to those problems. And that's what this book is all about.

Chapter one, *The Health Snapshot*, will help you to begin looking at your parent's health from a functional standpoint: what he or she can and cannot do for him or herself, what to expect in the future, and how a doctor can help fill in the blanks. You'll also learn everything from how to schedule lunch-hour telephone consultations to where to get free pamphlets on senior nutrition and health aids. Follow this step-by-step guide and by the end of chapter one, you'll be operating from a position of strength.

In chapter two, *Modifying the Home Environment*, You'll find dozens of fast, easy ways to make your parent's home safer and more convenient. You'll learn more than just how to accident-proof the home: we'll guide you on a weekend room-by-room analysis of what to move, lower, tie up, install or remove. By the end of chapter two, you'll have a list of suggested equipment and gadgets to acquire, and you'll know where to buy them for less or how to make them yourself.

Chapter three, *Where to Get Help*, is a guided tour through the elder care network. Here you'll learn where to find free and low-cost help—everything from dollar-a-ride medical vans that will take Mom to the doctor, to home-delivered meals, to drug stores that deliver, to the bookmobile. We'll teach you to find the best paid services and get into free programs. By the end of this chapter, you'll have a custom-designed plan for your parent.

In chapter four, *Balancing Caregiving and the Workplace*, you'll learn how to re-structure your workday and caregiving routines and eliminate the deadwood. Here, we'll be looking at ways to get more done in less time. You'll also find out how to talk to your boss—what to say and what not to say, how to arrange for emergency time off, and how to reduce caregiving-related absences. You don't have to pass up that promotion—you just have to put these timesavers to work.

Chapter five, *Long-Distance Caregiving*, is full of practical help for long-distance caregivers. Use these suggestions and techniques to set up the caregiving network via telephone, fax and mail. Learn how to screen out substandard service providers, hire a home health aide from 1,000 miles away and appoint an in-town overseer. This chapter will make emergency trips and sleepless nights the exception rather than the rule.

Now you're ready to go over your parent's financial and legal affairs. Chapter six, *Legal and Financial Issues* covers such considerations as consolidating bank accounts, to why Mom needs a medical power of attorney, to nursing home insurance and Medicare. Along the way, you'll find out how Mom can pay for home health care with her house equity, and see how one toll-free telephone call can get her monthly Social Security checks deposited directly into the bank.

In chapter seven, *Hands-on Caregiving Techniques*, you'll learn such basics as how to lift Mom, how to make a bed while she's in it, and helpful personal care tips. You'll become familiar with common age-related conditions and learn to identify potential medical problems.

Chapter eight, *Caring for You, The Caregiver*, is all about you. It's full of easy, practical suggestions and techniques to help you reduce stress and focus on your own needs. Learn to set limits for yourself and regain mental, emotional and physical equilibrium.

For the sake of convenience, the text switches back and forth between genders (he, she) and parental titles (Mom to Dad).

At the end of each chapter we have included creative "Timesavers" as well as a short "To Do This Week" list that'll get you moving in a positive direction. In the back of the book you'll find dozens of resources, most with toll-free telephone numbers. It is here that you'll find everthing from where to order custom-designed adult diapers to caregiver support groups.

. . . .

Caring for Your Aging Parents is your no-nonsense, quick-and-easy trail map through the caregiving wilderness.
Now, let's get started.

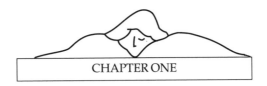

CHAPTER ONE

THE HEALTH SNAPSHOT

. . . .

"One afternoon while I was at work, Dad collapsed in the backyard. At the hospital, the doctor asked me if Dad was following the salt-restricted, fluid-restricted diet prescribed "to prevent this episode of congestive heart failure." I was blown away. He'd been going for dialysis three times a week, but he never said anything about heart failure or a special diet—and just a few days before, I'd taken over a honey-baked ham. We'd sat on the patio and drank a pitcher of lemonade while we ate it. He's 80 years old now, and I guess he didn't want to face his health problems. And there I was, ignorant, feeding him ham and lemonade."

—Dorothy, office manager, age 50

FOR MOST WORKING CAREGIVERS, THE HARDEST THING IS LEARNing to intervene gracefully and appropriately in a parent's life. For instance, Dad may appreciate having help with the laundry but bristle when you ask if his finances are okay. And how many of us want to give up our driver's license?

Caregiving isn't about taking control of another person's life. Although the tone of this book may seem to encourage aggressive intervention, we're just trying to cover all the bases for caregivers whose parents are extremely impaired either physically or mentally.

So as you read, adapt the suggestions to fit the needs, abilities and desires of your loved ones as well as of yourself. By a process of trial and error, you'll learn what types of assistance you can give Dad that will leave his self-respect and personal autonomy intact.

As a caregiver, it is essential that you know what's going on with your parent physically, mentally and emotionally. Acquiring such knowledge requires some detective work on your part, along with input from your parent and his physicians, including the internist, ophthalmologist and cardiologist.

STARTING YOUR NOTEBOOK

First, buy an inexpensive three-ring notebook. Pick a notebook that's large and can accommodate lots of papers. You'll also want to get some notebook paper and a couple of ringed folders to hold loose papers and pamphlets.

For added convenience, divide the notebook into four or five sections, using tabbed dividers. On each tab, write the contents of that section. For example, you might divide your notebook into "health info," "housing," "providers," "financial/legal," and "to-do lists and calendar."

Use this notebook to consolidate records and materials, track caregiving tasks and keep yourself organized. Carry it with you. Record telephone numbers, dates and important deadlines or conversations in it. If you use the notebook properly, you'll actually be writing your own caregiving manual!

GATHERING HEALTH INFORMATION

The next step is to find a quiet place where you don't have to worry about being disturbed, and have a talk with Dad. If he's experiencing any physical, mental or emotional problems, record them in your notebook. Does he walk with difficulty? Does he forget to feed the dog? Does he talk about feeling lonely or useless? Is he too frail to mow the lawn? Has he given up painting since the stroke made his right side weak? Is he able to feed himself?

Now add any problems you suspect but aren't sure of. Is he bathing less because of a frightening fall in the bathtub? Does he seem more disoriented since switching to the new blood pressure medicine? Does he discourage visits from friends because he feels depressed?

With notebook in hand, sit down and talk to Dad. You'll want to find out everything you can about his family history here: Did his father have heart problems too? Did any of his aunts or uncles suffer from strokes or cancer? Ask him what the doctor said about his current health status. Is he anemic or hypertensive? How long before the worst effects of the stroke will pass? Is he taking his medications as prescribed by the doctor? Does he seem evasive or say things like "that doctor doesn't know what she's talking about"?

Now steer the conversation toward his emotional well-being. How is Dad occupying himself while you're at work? Is he watching TV all day? Has arthritis forced him to give up his weekly bridge games? Has he quit going to church since he gave up driving? Do any friends call or visit? Has a special pet died recently? Would he consider adopting a new friend from the animal pound? Does he have trouble sleeping?

Line up his pill bottles on the kitchen table. Don't forget to include over-the-counter remedies like laxatives and aspirin. On a separate page, write down each medication, along with the prescribed dosage, instructions and doctor's name. Be sure to write down the name, address and telephone number of the drugstore where he gets the prescriptions filled so that such information is available for future use.

Go over any insurance policies or medical bills with him, if possible. Is he on Medicare or Medicaid? Is he still covered by an employer-sponsored health plan, or has he bought a private policy? Does he have nursing home insurance? Do any of the policies cover home health care or prescription drugs? In the notebook, write down Dad's social security number, Medicare or Medicaid I.D. number, or insurance plan number. Check the bills for any "claim assistance" telephone numbers and write them down, too.

Use a sixth page to evaluate any adaptive devices he's using. Does he wear a hearing aid? Is it working properly? How long has it been since he visited the audiologist for a check up or hearing-aid adjustment? Hearing technology is changing rapidly, and he may be able to hear better by switching to a more recent model.

Does he wear glasses? Bifocals? When was his last visit to the ophthalmologist? Has he given up reading as his eyesight worsened? Has he tried reading with the assistance of a print magnifier? Do his glasses rub his nose and cause blisters or soreness?

Is his walker adjusted properly for his height, or does he have to bend way over to use it? Can he move his wheelchair easily, or would a more lightweight model be better? Does his surgical corset pinch and cause skin irritations? Does he wear adult diapers or elastic stockings?

Be sure to write down the names, addresses and telephone numbers of his ophthalmologist, audiologist, or medical supply company for future reference.

TALKING WITH THE DOCTOR

This is a good time to ask Dad if he'd like you to accompany him on his next medical appointment. If you feel more immediate and direct intervention is appropriate, then call Dad's primary physician. Ask the nurse when the doctor is available for a telephone consultation. If possible, schedule your lunch hour so you'll be free to speak to the doctor from work.

Introduce yourself to the doctor, and explain that you're acting as your father's caregiver. Some doctors will refuse to discuss a patient's health without written consent from the patient, so you may need to have your father write the doctor a letter of permission on your behalf.

Ask the doctor about Dad's physical health. Has he been diagnosed with a specific condition or disease? What is the future prognosis for each condition? For instance, if he's recovering from a stroke, you might ask:

✓ How has the stroke affected Dad's muscular strength or neurological functioning? Would a hand brace (or other assistive eating device) help him maneuver a fork and knife better? Should you feed him, or encourage him to start feeding himself?

✓ What side effects does each prescribed medication have? Could Dad switch to a cheaper generic equivalent? How long will he have to take each medication? Do any of the medications on your page interact badly with each other? Read over the instructions for each medication and be sure to check that Dad is taking the medication as directed.

✓ Given your work schedule and Dad's current health status, does the doctor recommend hiring a home health assistant or companion? Does he make referrals to home health care companies?

✓ How long will Dad need speech, physical or occupational therapy? Can you help Dad do range of motion exercises? Can the doctor recommend a therapist who makes house calls, or can teach you to do range-of-motion exercises? Should you take Dad for short walks? Does he have any physical limitations?

✓ Should you buy a shower chair? Or start pricing wheelchairs? Do you need to buy an adjustable bed? Does the doctor deal with a specific medical supply house? Can he write a medical prescription for any of the equipment for insurance purposes?

Be sure to share your notebook observations with the doctor. He needs to know if Dad is depressed, not taking his heart medication regularly, or experiencing shortness of breath.

Ask the doctor or his medical social worker for lists of service providers and community resources—home health care companies, medical supply houses, adult daycare programs, insurance paperwork assistance programs, respite caregivers, caregiver support groups (more on this in chapters 4, 5 and 6). Also ask for any written information—fact sheets, sample meal plans, do's and don'ts—that he gives to patients.

If Dad recently had a physical examination, you and the doctor should be able to pool information and come up with a definitive health "snapshot." If not, consider scheduling an exam for Dad for late afternoon or early morning, and take a couple hours off work to go along. Talk with the doctor before and after the exam, and take your notebook along to write everything down.

While most doctors are happy to oblige their patients and caregivers, some don't take the time to deal with questions. Many doctors employ social workers for just this purpose—to interact with patients, answer questions and troubleshoot.

What if you feel a doctor is not treating Dad's health with the proper concern? You might want to offer assistance; perhaps Dad would like to find another physician. Many hospitals have physician-referral telephone services. You may also want to ask friends and coworkers for names of good physicians.

. . . .

Now that you and Dad have a clear idea of his health status, things will go much smoother. He knows you'll help in whatever ways he considers appropriate. You've discovered important facts about his health status and life-style. You will both have a better idea as to what to expect in the future. You've also taken the first step in improving Dad's daily comfort level— and reducing your own stress level.

✓

Utilize your "fringe time." Get up early and run a caregiving errand on the way to work. Check in with Dad via telephone during your lunch hour and during breaks, or use lunches for caregiving telephone calls to doctors and service providers.

✓

Whenever possible, ask to have information—catalogues, company brochures, price lists and application forms—mailed to you.

✓

Write everything down in your notebook. When you speak to a doctor, pharmacist, medical social worker, insurance company or Medicare representative, note the time, date, their name and title, and what they said. Carry the notebook to work with you, so you will have telephone numbers and information at your fingertips. Cross "to do" items off once each task is completed so you don't get behind or forget something important.

✓

Buy an inexpensive calendar—the kind you hang over your desk. Punch holes in it with a hole puncher, and put it in the back of your notebook. Use it to keep track of doctor appointments and medication refills.

✓

Order the free pamphlet called "Healthy Older People" from the National Health Information Center, U.S. Department of Health and Human Services, P.O. Box 1133, Washington, DC 20012, telephone (800) 336-4797. Ask to receive "Staying Healthy," a list of free government health publications.

✓

Call local pharmacies and ask if they deliver free to elderly clients. Compare drug prices by phone, and then ask Dad if he'd like to have his prescriptions transferred to the best store. Switch your own prescriptions to the same store. You may also want to check into mail-order pharmaceutical companies, or patronize a pharmacy within walking distance of your office.

✓

Call the local library's reference desk and ask them to reserve books on caregiving or a specific medical condition in your name, and pick the books up on your way home from work. If Dad seems interested, see if a bookmobile visits his neighborhood: they may also have large-size print books and books on tape cassettes. Some libraries even loan out tape recorders to seniors.

✓

Call local bookstores and ask if they stock large-print books or books on tape cassettes. Do they have publishers' catalogues you can review? For serious visual impairments, call the American Foundation for the Blind, Inc. at (800) 232-5463 for a free catalog of products including watches, clocks, calculators, canes and other items.

✓

If Dad has a serious hearing impairment, call the AT&T National Special Needs Center, (800) 233-1222, or (800) 233-3232 TDD. Their free catalog includes a helpful variety of wonderful adaptive equipment—emergency call systems, telephone amplifiers, and more.

✓

Call 1-800-521-0097 to order a free catalogue called "Comfortably Yours." It is there you will find reasonably priced gadgets such as back-pampering snow shovels, amplifying telephones, wrist watches with oversized numbers, custom incontinence products, and a spectacular "long arm" device that helps a seated person pick things up off the floor.

✓

Check with local grocery stores, too—many of them deliver free to seniors. Ask to have order forms and catalogues mailed to you.

✓

If Dad is not sure what his insurance policy covers, give his agent a call to review coverages, deductibles, matching fees, exclusions and waiting periods. If necessary, ask the agent to come to your workplace during the lunch hour to discuss the policy, or meet with both you and Dad at Dad's home.

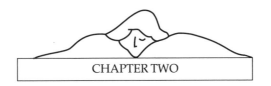

CHAPTER TWO

MODIFYING THE HOME ENVIRONMENT

· · · · · · · · ·

"We call my mother-in-law's electric wheelchair 'Mom's Roommate.' Because of her new roommate, all kinds of changes had to be made. Ramps to the front and back door. Door frames widened. She had to buy a new recliner, because she couldn't get herself in and out of the wheelchair into the old one—the recliner arms were in the way. Everything changes when you can't walk. We moved her bedroom from upstairs to the formal dining room, which seems odd to some of our guests, I'm sure, but she can be in the middle of the family ebb and flow this way. We serve guests dinner in the family room instead. We saved money by making a lot of things ourselves, too, and renting the big items like the wheelchair and the hoist."

—*Helen, secretary, age 46*

CAREGIVING IS EASIER WHEN YOUR PARENT HAS A SAFE, ACCESsible living environment. In some cases, a move to a groundfloor apartment or an assisted living community may be necessary. But with a little work, most people can stay in their own home.

Set aside a weekend afternoon for a walking tour of Mom's home. Bring along the notebook and write down your observations and her comments. Whenever possible, involve your mother in this process. Her input is extremely important, since she knows which aspects of her living environment pose the greatest barriers. Ask her what changes she would like made.

Start with the basic layout of the home. Your goal is to customize the house or apartment to Mom's current and future needs, so be creative and think ahead.

TRADING PLACES

Try an easy experiment: put yourself in your mother's place for an hour or two. If she has a wheelchair, get in it, and see if you can reach the light switches or thermostat. Try to swing yourself from the wheelchair to the toilet. Would "grab bars" around the toilet or tub help you maneuver more easily? Imagine someone knocking on the front door—is the peephole in the door too high to see through? Peephole kits are cheap and easy to install.

Take Mom's walker into the kitchen. While keeping one hand on the walker, are you able to operate the electric can opener? Can you reach into overhead cabinets without losing your balance? Now put an unopened can of soup in a saucepan. Using the walker, try to carry the pan to the kitchen table. How hard is it to wash dishes, put a new liner in the trash can, or bend over to feed the cat?

Is furniture arranged for easy passage? Are there dangling electrical cords Mom could trip over or low-hanging plants that are difficult to water? Do doors need to be widened for her wheelchair? Can steps be covered with ramps, and railings installed? Consider covering elevated door sills with ramps and installing handrails in hallways.

Shag or thick carpets are harder to walk on than flat carpeting or bare floors. Slick, waxed floors and scatter rugs can be dangerous, too. Many discount stores carry nonskid rug liners in various shapes, or rolls that can be cut to conform to any rug's shape. Be sure Mom has nonskid slippers or shoes to wear around the house.

Poor lighting can lead to falls. Many people find that buying higher-wattage light bulbs does the trick. And check the water heater—if it's set too high, Mom can scald herself.

You may want to replace a wall-mounted telephone with a handset telephone. Program emergency numbers into the telephone, as well as a friendly neighbor's number and your home and work numbers.

How about a cordless telephone? If Mom is hard of hearing, buy a telephone amplifier or turn the telephone ringer to the highest setting. You can also buy a device that turns on a lamp whenever the telephone rings, alerting her to an incoming call. If her eyesight or hand-eye coordination is bad, shop for a special telephone that has extra-large numerical buttons on the face.

If Mom has trouble turning doorknobs, replace them with lever-style handles. You can also buy inexpensive glow-in-the dark doorknob covers to help her get around at night.

Some seniors feel safer once they install a security system, while others find them a bother. Check doors and windows: if they don't have easy-to-use locks, visit a hardware store and check out the newest models. Doors should have dead bolts.

Window (security) bars should be the inside, swing-open type, in case Mom needs to get out during a fire. Plan an emergency escape route from a large window, and station a step stool underneath it so she can climb out, if necessary.

The home should also have at least one smoke detector (check batteries regularly) and a lightweight fire extinguisher stored where it's easy to grab. Go over the instructions with her so she knows how to use the fire extinguisher. Check with the fire department to be sure Mom's home complies to fire safety guidelines. Make sure she has a lightweight flashlight handy for power outages. Select a flashlight that is easy for her to operate (some are too heavy for seniors or are difficult to turn on and off).

Here are some additional possibilities to consider:

BATHROOM

- Replace bathtub/shower glass doors with a shower curtain for easy access.
- Replace a "spring rod" with a screw-in shower curtain rod —if Mom starts to fall and grabs the shower curtain, the screw-in rod will offer more support.
- Install metal "grab bars" around the toilet and bathtub/shower.
- Buy a shower chair or bench so Mom can sit comfortably and climb in and out safely.
- Install an inexpensive hand-held shower attachment so Mom can wash her hair while sitting.
- Put adhesive nonslip strips on the bottom of the tub/shower to prevent falls.
- Clearly mark the water faucets as "hot" and "cold."
- How about an "emergency call" button for the bathroom?
- Get an adjustable-height stool or chair so Mom can brush her teeth and hair while sitting down. Have her sit on it while you adjust the height so that she can see herself in the bathroom mirror.

KITCHEN

- Put appliances—toaster, can opener, coffee maker, hot plate, microwave, toaster oven—on a table, adjusted for easy operation from a wheelchair or regular kitchen chair. Put pet food dishes and supplies on another, smaller table to make bending over less of a problem.
- Rearrange kitchen cabinets and drawers so that supplies and items used daily are easy to reach. If Mom has some memory impairment, clearly label cupboards and drawers—"Canned Food" or "Plates," for instance.
- If Mom is unsteady, buy some nonbreakable glasses and dishes in bright colors and pretty patterns.
- Keep things out instead of putting them away. Screw large cup hooks into a wall low enough to reach: hang hot pads,

pans, a colander, and utensils on them. Some kitchen stores sell attractive plastic-coated wire grids for this purpose.

- If a spice rack is in a high cabinet or hanging over the stove, move it lower.
- Modify kitchen utensils so that handles are enlarged and easier to grab. Try wrapping handles with foam rubber topped with electrical tape.
- Buy a simple "reacher" device to help get out-of-the-way items down from cupboards.
- Again, an adjustable, wheeled stool or chair can make food preparation and cleanup easier and can be wheeled between stove, counter, table and sink.

BEDROOM

- Lower or raise the bed so Mom can get in and out easily. Price water beds, air mattresses or foam pads for extra comfort and to prevent bedsores. You may want to rent or buy an electric or manual hospital bed, or install side rails on a regular bed.
- Shop the medical supply house for a mechanical hoist if Mom is too heavy to lift out of bed into a wheelchair, or buy an over-the-bed trapeze to help her move around in bed.
- How about an over-the-bed table like those used in hospitals? Mom can then write letters, read a book, play solitaire or eat comfortably this way. The same type of table can also be used with a wheelchair during the daytime hours.
- Buy a commode chair or bedpan for nighttime emergencies.
- Be sure to have a telephone programmed with emergency numbers within easy reach of the bed, preferably on a bedside table.
- Buy an inexpensive clock with large, easy-to-see numbers for the bedside table, a clock that projects the time on the ceiling or a "talking" clock.

- Keep a plastic pitcher, cup and lightweight flashlight on the bedside table so Mom won't have to get up for a drink of water at night.
- If there are problems with incontinence, buy a couple of plastic mattress covers, and layer a mattress pad on top for comfort and to prevent slipping.
- Plug in simple night lights throughout the house—in the hallway, bathroom, kitchen and bedroom.

LIVING ROOM
- Check with an electronics store for remote-control devices for her television, VCR and stereo.
- Experiment with a "clap on" device for light switches.
- Price adjustable chairs or "lift" chairs.
- Keep small pillows and an afghan in reach for napping in chairs or on the couch. Lumbar cushions are helpful for people with back problems.
- Wedge cushions can help keep Mom upright and comfortable in a wheelchair, as can a Velcro, self-releasing wheelchair "seat belt."
- Keep extra-large playing cards, large-size print paperback books or large-size print crossword puzzle books in easy reach of the chair.
- Have cable installed on the television to provide a wide range of viewing choices.
- Buy a lightweight tape recorder or an inexpensive radio so Mom can listen to music.
- How about a lightweight, clip-on fan for a chair-side table or wheelchair arm?
- To raise a sofa or easy chair (for easier in-and-out), nail wooden four-by-fours to the furniture base.

OUTDOORS
- Install ramps over stairs or install handrails.

- If finances permit, hire a neighborhood teen to take over lawn mowing, weeding and snow shoveling, or hire a landscaping service to do everything from fertilizing to tree trimming.
- Install an automated watering system, or pay a neighborhood child to water as necessary.
- Store a bag of rock salt by the front door during winter and keep a scoop in it so Mom can throw salt on any ice on the doorstep.
- Make gardening easier. Buy a gardening stool or foam knee pad. Burpee and other garden tool manufacturers sell special long-handled tools for seniors. Wrap tool handles with foam padding topped with tape.
- Replace water-greedy flower beds and lawns with xeriscaping (low-water landscaping). Your water department or nursery can recommend beautiful trees, bushes, ground cover, grass and flowers that require very little maintenance. Or consider replacing a lawn with a rock garden or cactus.
- Instead of a vegetable garden, plant a few pots with tomatoes, carrots or sweet-smelling flowers.

WHAT YOU NEED

Make a "wish list" of remodeling projects and things to buy or rent, along with a list of things you can make or rig up. Enlist the help of friends, family, neighbors and coworkers. For instance, divide shopping chores among siblings, ask your carpenter friend to build a ramp, and invite neighbors over one weekend afternoon to help winterize the house.

. . . .

Things will go more smoothly once Mom's home environment is modified. She will be living in a safer, more convenient environment, and you'll have fewer emergencies to cope with as a result.

✓

Physical therapists, hospital discharge planners and medical social workers may have tips on how to modify a home environment. They are also familiar with gadgets that help elderly people, so give them a call. Ask for names of reputable suppliers and have any written materials mailed to you.

✓

Check with Medicare or the insurance agent to see what items might be covered by either plan before making any significant purchases.

✓

Before spending lots of money, call your local hardware store and explain what you need. They might have something that will fill the bill for less money than a medical supply house.

✓

Call the local Area Agency on Aging. Funded by the Older Americans Act, AAAs operate in every county in the United States. AAAs contract with local service agencies to provide help to seniors free or for a nominal cost. Call them for home repairs, maintenance and remodeling needs (more on this in chapter 3).

✓

Make a lunchtime call to the Better Business Bureau to check the track records of any professional services that you are considering.

✓

Order a brochure called "Making the Home Safer and More Convenient" from Kelly Assisted Living, Dept. GH, P.O. Box 331180, Detroit, MI 48232-7180.

✓

Order the "DoAble, Renewable Home" from the American Association of Retired Persons, 601 E Street N.W., Washington, DC 20049, for tips on adapting the home environment.

✓

Visit a medical supply house on your way home from work. Take along your notebook and wish list. Check into renting versus buying expensive equipment, or consider buying used equipment. Ask about payment plans, Medicare reimbursement, insurance filing and delivery charges.

✓

Use a couple of lunch hours to shop for Mom. Visit the dime store, kitchen store or hardware store with your wish list.

✓

Call your local Red Cross or Salvation Army. They may have used wheelchairs, walkers or other equipment available.

✓

Check the newspaper or call a local senior center for referrals to professionals who do home-remodeling work for reasonable rates. Many corporations and community service agencies do free repairs and maintenance for seniors, too (more on this in chapter 3).

CHAPTER THREE

WHERE TO GET HELP

· · · · · · · · ·

"I was working all day, then driving over to Mom's before and after work to cook, clean, do laundry, bathe her and get her into bed. By the time I got home, I was a basket case. My husband took a friend to fill my seat at football games.

"I was too tired for sex, too angry to be rational about everyday work problems, and feeling too guilty to ask for help. Then my chest pains started, and a friend forced me to the telephone.

"I didn't realize that there was such a thing as respite caregivers who would come and help me. And I thought Meals-on-Wheels were poison. Well, they're not fine cuisine, but Mom is a trooper. And now I have a life again."

— *Joyce, teacher, age 48*

NO ONE CAN, OR SHOULD, TAKE CARE OF ANOTHER PERSON without help. Here are three important sources for finding help:

✓ government/community agencies
✓ medical facilities and businesses catering to older people and caregivers
✓ relatives, friends, coworkers and neighbors

These sources make up the formal (agencies and businesses) and informal (private individuals) aging-services network. Use the telephone, Blue Pages (government listings) and Yellow Pages to hone in on your local network.

Identify which of your parent's urgent needs pose a problem. Take into consideration which needs you don't have the time, money, expertise or energy to meet. Use a separate page in your notebook for each need.

Each time you speak with an agency, business or private individual who might be able to help you, record the information in your notebook. Be sure to write down each program's eligibility criteria, along with documentation needed to prove eligibility and any deadlines or other important items.

GOVERNMENT/COMMUNITY SERVICES

Begin by calling the local Area Agency on Aging (AAA); check the telephone book for the one in your area. If nothing is listed under "Area Agency on Aging," make a quick call to the social services department. In some areas, the AAAs go by slightly different names.

AAA offices coordinate services for low-income or disabled seniors, using money set aside by the federal Older Americans Act. Most AAAs don't actually get into the caregiving business; instead, they contract with local companies or agencies to provide home-delivered meals, rides to doctor appointments, legal assistance and other services to seniors in each county.

Tell the AAA representative what problems you and Mom are facing. The representative will explain how you can access each service—who to contact and where to apply.

Next, call the social services department. Start with the city social services department, then check with the county and state offices. Again, ask about available services and eligibility requirements. You might also contact the local regional office of the U.S. Administration on Aging.

You can branch out into the rest of the aging services network. Every area network is different, but here are some possibilities:

- Red Cross
- Volunteers of America
- Public Bus System
- Veterans of Foreign Wars
- Medicare & Medicaid
- Housing Administration
- City & County Hospitals
- Health Fairs
- Utility Companies
- Local Senior/Recreation Centers
- Widowed Men and Women of America
- Senior Health Centers
- Food Stamps and Food Commodities
- Local Senior Advocacy Groups

- United Way
- Legal Aid Society
- Welfare
- Veteran's Administration
- Social Security
- Older Women's League
- Caregiver Support Groups
- Public Health Department

What can you expect from the above agencies? Here are some examples of services that are provided:

✓ Some Red Cross offices train adult volunteers to handle correspondence and bill-paying for vision-impaired seniors.

✓ The public health department often gives seniors free flu shots, and may have a nurse who makes house calls.

✓ The public bus system may have weekly neighborhood pickups for seniors needing a ride to local grocery stores.

✓ Health fairs, often held in indoor shopping malls, offer free diagnostic screenings for everything from diabetes to colon cancer.

✓ Utility companies (telephone, water, gas and electric providers) often offer discounts to needy seniors.

✓ Housing administrations offer discounted apartments to low-income seniors.

✓ Some organizations—including the Alzheimer's Association and the Older Women's League—may train volunteers as respite caregivers.
✓ Medicare and Medicaid, besides providing basic health care, may pay for health-related services and equipment.
✓ United Way offers "information and referral" service free to anyone who calls with a question.

Most communities have food banks, and some even have clothing or furniture banks. Some food banks have "senior day," when older people are welcome to take their time selecting groceries. And an elderly person may qualify for food stamps or government food commodities.

HEALTH FACILITIES AND BUSINESSES

Check into the local recreation centers and senior centers. Many offer specialized water aerobics, stretching, wheelchair dance or even walking clubs. They may sponsor bingo nights, bridge and pinochle games or Saturday pottery classes. Center employees may lead slow-paced nature walks or movie nights for seniors. If Mom enjoys something that's not on the activity schedule, talk to the activity director about making a change.

Many professional organizations volunteer their time and expertise to older people. Your local real estate association may host annual "fix up" weekends for seniors who need home repairs.

Check the telephone book for other groups that might assist seniors with a specific problem. For instance, an optometry association may have funds for low-income seniors who can't afford bifocals, or members of a dental association may manufacture dentures.

Some hospitals also offer free "ask-a-nurse" telephone lines and doctor referral services. Many hospitals are starting "senior clinics" staffed with doctors, nurses and social workers experienced in geriatric medicine. Some offer discounted prices for needy seniors. There may even be a government-subsidized adult day care program in your community.

There are probably several businesses in your area that serve seniors and their caregivers on a commercial basis. Take a look at the following Need/Service matchup for some ideas; then draw up your own. The prices mentioned below were gathered from service providers in Denver, Colorado, in late 1991. (Note: Prices may vary widely in different areas, and can change over time.)

TROUBLESHOOTING
Mom can't feed or dress herself, or is lonely.
- Home Health Care Company—home care assistant hired for two-hour morning shift; cost approximately $26 a day. Companion hired for slightly less.

Mom can't walk the dog.
- Animal Boarding/Veterinarian—"walker" hired to exercise the dog, cost approximately $7 a day. Mobile veterinarian makes house calls.

Mom can't clean or do laundry.
- Housekeeping Agency—maid/laundress hired for four hours a week; cost approximately $60 a week.

Mom can't cook.
- Professional Rent-A-Cooks—cook hired to prepare a week's worth of dinners in Mom's kitchen; cost approximately $50 a week.

Mom needs haircuts, manicures.
- Beauty Salon—licensed hairdresser or nail technician hired for weekly visit; cost approximately $30 for haircut and manicure.

Mom can't mow the lawn, trim trees, or shovel snow.
- Yard Maintenance Firm—yard assistant hired to care for outside as needed. May also install storm windows, do simple repair; cost approximately $13 an hour.

Mom needs daily injections or physical therapy.
- Home Health Care Company—professional nurse or therapist hired as needed, cost approximately $25 an hour. (Some home health care is covered by Medicare.)

Mom's affairs are a mess.
- Elder Care Case Managers—attorneys, social workers, nurses, and insurance agents specializing in senior needs are available; cost varies.

Mom can't stay alone while you're at work.
- Adult Day Care—pay for Mom to do crafts, take walks, and socialize with other seniors; cost approximately $30 a day.

Mom has trouble sleeping and you work the night shift.
- Home Health Care Company—hire a "sleep over" companion willing to get up when Mom's restless; cost approximately $12 an hour.

Before hiring someone to come into an elderly person's home, be sure to ask for references, and check the firm's track record with the Better Business Bureau.

Adult day care is a relatively new option. If there is a day care facility in your community, ask if Mom can spend a day there free of charge to see if she's comfortable in the environment. Drop in unannounced to see how well the staff cares for guests. Be sure to choose a facility with a dietician/nutritionist on staff, as well as an activity director and appropriate nursing professionals. Check the physical environment for safety and comfort.

Also, many businesses will deliver or make home-service calls for seniors. These same companies—medical supply houses, grocery stores, pharmacies—usually offer senior citizen discounts. Don't be afraid to ask for delivery or special service. For instance, many pet food stores will deliver to seniors for free. Grocery stores will cut up a watermelon or split a roast in half for senior customers.

THE INFORMAL NETWORK

What about help from the informal network—neighbors, friends, coworkers and relatives? Here are some ideas:

Friendly, concerned neighbors often want to help caregivers. Seniors living alone can be very vulnerable, so be careful who you ask for help. If neighbors offer—and after checking with Mom—you might ask them to:

✓ stop by Mom's on their way to the store; maybe she needs milk, or would like to go along;

✓ stop by or call to make sure Mom is okay;

✓ invite Mom the next time they barbecue in the backyard;

✓ keep a watchful eye out for strangers or burglars; or

✓ keep your work and home telephone numbers, as well as the number of Mom's doctor, posted by their telephone.

You might also consider hiring a trustworthy neighborhood child to walk Mom's dog or do yard work. If a neighbor cares for young children during the day, maybe she would include Mom on walks or visits to the park for a small fee.

Are there Boy Scouts in Mom's neighborhood? Some troops shovel snow for seniors free of charge. How about the local homeowners association? Do they tackle projects—like painting or insulating attics—for needy seniors?

Many churches or synagogues have clergy and volunteers who deliver food baskets or visit lonely seniors. Church-goers who live near Mom might take turns picking her up for Sunday services or potlucks. Attend church with her so you can meet these people, and offer them your telephone number. Check the activity calendar—is there a senior's knitting circle, bible study or bingo night Mom would enjoy? Can you drop her off or ask a church-goer to pick up Mom?

DON'T GO IT ALONE!

It's tough, but not impossible, to involve other relatives in Mom's caregiving. Typically, one or two persons, usually adult daughters, will shoulder the majority of the caregiving work, only to become resentful and unhappy because they are over-whelmed by the emotional stress and physical work.

So how do you involve other relatives? First, don't act as if you and you alone are responsible for Mom. If relatives offer to help out, don't turn them down; if they don't offer, don't be afraid to ask for their help. Let them know that together, you can build a network of helpers. Call a family meeting to review Mom's needs and encourage each person's input. Help relatives choose caregiving tasks according to each person's schedule, activities and interests. For instance, does your college-age son spend hours in the library? Ask him to pick up and drop off library books for Mom. Give him a list of authors to get started, and encourage him to look around for interesting-looking books. Or do you have a daughter-in-law who works in a grocery store? Give her Mom's shopping list. Does your son work in construction? Ask him to be Mom's handyman. Is your sister a banker? Ask her to look over Mom's financial affairs.

Encourage relatives to visit Mom, and include her in their daily lives. Do both your husband and Mom love garage-sale excursions? Invite Mom along, and start out early in the day before she tires or it gets too warm. Do Mom's sisters take daily constitutionals around the neighborhood? Maybe one day a week they can include her, and walk a little slower.

If Mom likes to go places but needs to take along gear—adult diapers, blood sugar testers and syringes, medication, a sweater—buy an inexpensive backpack and keep it packed.

Whoever picks up Mom just has to grab the pack and insert her purse and keys.

Is Mom's house on anyone's way home from work or school? Ask each person to stop by to visit and perform a task once or twice a week. For instance, Marie could fix dinner for Mom on Tuesdays and Thursdays, Bob could do a load of wash on Mondays and Wednesdays, and Aunt Martha could take Mom to the store Friday evenings. Grandchildren can share a Saturday matinee movie with Mom. A niece attending nursing school may want to help Mom with her physical therapy.

Do you or relatives belong to a group such as the Elks, Kiwanis, Rotary Club, Jaycees, Eastern Star, church or synagogue? Does the group sponsor needy seniors? Would they consider holding a bake sale to raise money for Mom's adjustable hospital bed? Does anyone in the group do low-cost home repairs?

Many of your coworkers have aging parents, too. Can you link up for fun and convenience? How about getting tickets to see a play after work with your respective parents? Or split lunch-hour trips to the pharmacy—you pick up their prescriptions one day, they get yours next time. Call the local branch of the AARP to find out when the next "caregiving fair" will be held, and then ask a coworker if they'd like to come, too. Does your coworker know of a good adult day care center, a trustworthy yard boy, or a home health agency?

. . . .

*Some of your hardest work as a working caregiver is now
accomplished. You've drawn together resources from your
community into a caregiving network. Next we'll look
at how you can make your on-the-job time easier.*

✓

If you are unable to locate the AAA in your area, call the National Association of Area Agencies on Aging at (202) 484-7520 for assistance.

✓

When applying for government or community agencies, have all applications and guidelines mailed to you.

✓

Make multiple copies of documents commonly requested by government or community agencies—income statements and tax or medical records—so you'll have them handy.

✓

Keep copies of completed applications in your notebook so you won't have to start over if someone loses Mom's paperwork.

✓

Call Maddak, Inc. at (800) 443-4926 for a free catalog of "daily living aids" for seniors' recreation, transportation, grooming, home health care and rehab needs.

✓

If lunch-hour telephone calls aren't getting the job done, take half a day or a full day off to tie up loose ends, such as signing papers, interviewing home health care companies or presenting Mom for a preenrollment health assessment.

✓

Ask the AAA representative if there is a "seniors' service directory" available in your community. If so, have it mailed to your home.

✓

Stop by the neighborhood senior center on your lunch hour or on the way home from work. Check out the activities and staff, and bring home a schedule of events.

✓

Call the AARP's Pharmacy Service at (800) 456-2277 for a free catalog of prescription and over-the-counter drugs, vitamins, dental products and personal care items sold via the mail. You have to be a member to use the service, but AARP membership is under $10 annually.

✓

Get a subscription to the local newspaper for older people. These papers are great reading for Mom and a good resource guide for caregivers. (If you don't know where to find such a paper, ask the AAA representative.)

✓

Send for a consumer's guide to home health care from the National Association for Home Care, 519 C Street N.E., Stanton Park, Washington, DC 20002, or call (202) 547-7424.

✓

To find out what other services are available locally, contact the office of state and community programs at the U.S. Administration on Aging, 330 Independence Avenue S.W., Washington, DC 20201, or telephone (202) 619-0724.

✓

Begin an essential caregiver mental health ritual: no matter what must be put aside, spend a couple of hours with a friend, lover, spouse or a good book. Or tune in your favorite radio station and really participate—sing the blues, conduct the orchestra or wail about the man who got away—as you wash dishes, cook Mom's lunches for next week, pay bills or fold laundry for both households. You'll feel alive again.

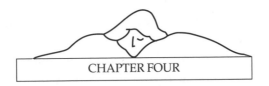

CHAPTER FOUR

BALANCING CAREGIVING AND THE WORKPLACE

· · · · · · · · ·

"My boss didn't understand what I was doing. His priority was that all employees get their work done, and that was that. The longer I took care of my mother-in-law, the harder that got. My husband still thought it was my responsibility, although this is *his* mother.

"So things got pretty bad at the station. I was late to work on mornings when Mother had wet the bed: I had to change and bathe her, get out new sheets, throw the wet ones in the washer and turn it on. I ran around her house with my teeth clenched. By 8:00 a.m. my head was splitting, and my boss would come over to me and say something snotty."

—*Caroline, television advertising sales, age 53*

IT'S NOT EASY TO BALANCE WORK WITH CAREGIVING AND FAMILY obligations. Often, caregivers have children or grandchildren of various ages to look after in addition to an elderly person.

Although you may enjoy your career, you probably work for one overwhelming reason: you need the money. Your job is also essential to your security, well-being and happiness. Since you probably can't afford to lose your job, it's important to find ways to handle caregiving and working. The most important thing is balance: between work and play, between caregiving and receiving care (more on "caring for the caregiver" in chapter 8), between your children and your parents.

One way to organize caregiving and working responsibilities is to use a page in your notebook to break down your job- and caregiving-related tasks and time constraints. Be sure to include probable overtime, as well as seasonal busy periods.

Here's how Caroline's job page read:

7:00 a.m. Get to Mother's house. Help her up, give her a quick bath if she's been incontinent overnight. Fix breakfast; help her dress; set up water pitcher, glass, snacks, TV guide, remote control and afghan by her chair; get her settled. Make sure something easy to fix is in the refrigerator or freezer. Get cats in house, lock up, leave for work.

8:00 a.m. Have to be at work. Mornings, call on advertisers in person. Can make caregiving-related calls from desk as long as secretary isn't backed up with my incoming calls.

Noon. One-hour lunch, which I often spend taking clients out to eat and making sales pitches.

Afternoons. Very busy. Daily 3:00 p.m. sales meetings lasting only half an hour. Weekly p.m. meetings with manager. Can't really receive personal calls. Have to push to get paperwork done, and can never leave by 5:00 p.m. During presweeps or preholiday periods, add at least two hours to my on-the-job time. During annual Jerry Lewis Telethon, have to work the telethon. Also, monthly meetings with the employee benefit committee. Sometimes go out for a much needed drink-and-whine session with coworkers. At least once every other week, need time off to take Mother to the doctor.

6:00 p.m. Leave work late. Do my own and Mother's grocery shopping, pick up prescriptions, go by her house on way home. Do a load of laundry, put away groceries, make her dinner, help her bathe and get ready for bed, clean kitchen.

8:00 p.m. Home to my husband and adult son, where they expect me to do the same chores for them that I did for Mother. To bed at midnight.

Weekends. Take Mother out for a drive and church on Sundays. Clean her house and my own, finish both laundries, do everything else. No time for me.

Let's look at ways Caroline might make her schedule easier to handle:

WORK TIME

✓ Take a half-day time management class. Many employers sponsor these, or will foot the bill for interested employees. Caroline needs to learn to prioritize tasks, organize paperwork and manage work flow.

✓ Quit working through lunch. Caroline can use the hour to get a haircut, eat at her desk and chat with friends by telephone, reorder Mother's prescriptions, or consult with Mother's doctor—without doing it on her employer's time.

✓ Use breaks to make caregiving telephone calls. Caroline should be specific about her time constraints and when her call can be returned. If the person she is trying to reach can't call back right away, she should ask the person to call during lunch.

✓ Since both the Jerry Lewis Telethon and the employee benefit committee are voluntary positions, Caroline should take a leave of absence or resign from these activities. This will mean less stress and more time to sell ads.

✓ Concentrate on arriving and leaving on time. During presweeps and preholiday periods, Caroline should hire respite caregivers, arrange for volunteers or recruit family and friends to fill in for her.

✓ Caroline should avoid complaining to coworkers about her difficult schedule as a working caregiver. People rarely keep a secret. That innocent revelation, "I've been getting four hours of sleep lately, so when old McPherson said to rework the report, I told *him*" could be a time bomb. Managers take such things into consideration when calculating raises, laying off employees and awarding promotions.

CAREGIVING TIME

✓ Switch some tasks from early morning to evening, when Caroline's husband and adult son can help out. For instance, lay out Mother's clothes, set the table and get her chairside items arranged before leaving at night.

✓ Don't let the cats out in the morning, if getting them back in the house is time consuming.

✓ Cut down on laundry by buying rubber mattress covers for under the bed sheets. Try using adult diapers or extra-large toddler diapers for added protection and to prevent skin rashes.

✓ Arrange for Mother to receive Meals-on-Wheels for lunch.

✓ Hire a home health assistant to fix dinner, do laundry and tidy the house, as well as help Mother bathe and get into bed. Estimated cost: $26 for two hours, three times a week equals $78.

✓ Switch to a grocery store and pharmacy that deliver to seniors free or for a small additional cost.

✓ Caroline should encourage her husband and son to take over or come along at least three nights a week, and also to help out at home. Anyone can sort clothes and operate a washer/dryer, rinse dishes and run a dishwasher, prepare simple meals or shop for groceries.

✓ Caroline's husband has two sisters and a brother who live nearby. Her husband should divide caregiving days with them, or assign on-the-way-home shopping and errand-running to each.

✓ Sign Mother up for free or low-cost rides to doctors' appointments through the local AAA, United Way or other agency so Caroline won't have to leave work to drive her.

✓ Ask about car pools and social outings for seniors at Mother's church or the local senior center. See about getting her involved in activities in order to free up Caroline's weekends and keep Mother happy.

✓ Schedule a completely "caregiving free" weekend every month. Let others handle the work and assign "backup emergency" to another family member.

TALKING TO THE BOSS

Sometimes the scale tips, though, and a crisis takes over. At what point should an employee discuss his or her caregiving obligations with management?

Be frank with your boss. If you suddenly need time off work to move Mother into another apartment, for instance, tell your boss the truth. Meet with him and explain the problem. Estimate the time you'll need and be back at work as scheduled. Put the terms of your time off in writing so there will be no disputes later about whether your time off constituted vacation time, sick leave, personal days, or simply time off that must be made up later.

If your work schedule is in direct conflict with Mother's caregiving needs, meet with an employee relations advisor. Ask about flex-time, job-sharing, cutting back to part-time, or switching from day to night shift.

Does your company have an Employee Assistance Program? If so, see if it can refer you to a good doctor or elder care counselor, or help you find a reputable home health care provider.

Don't lie to your employer. If you're caught doing so, it will mean embarrassment—and possibly worse. At the same time, don't reveal personal information that isn't essential at that moment.

Managers are human, and it will be hard for them to forget a comment like, "I'm so stressed out that I cry in the bathroom," when they write your performance review. Even if your job productivity hasn't been impacted by your caregiving duties, someone else might perceive that it was.

HARD CHOICES

Here's another working caregiver's dilemma: Julie's father was diagnosed with Alzheimer's disease soon after she was promoted to office manager. For two months, she struggled to care for him alone, even sleeping at his house several nights a week. She couldn't afford to hire a respite caregiver, so when he started wandering away at night, she moved in.

At the same time, her job responsibilities increased so that she was spending ten hours a day at the office. A new branch manager arrived and began complaining when Julie said she couldn't stay for his early-evening meetings. A coworker circulated rumors about her "crazy father," and hinted that Julie wasn't capable of handling her job.

The coworker was partly right. The new branch manager did expect at least ten hours of work a day from Julie, and she could no longer comply with such an expectation. She met with him and proposed that someone else be appointed office manager, and volunteered to resume her position as billings clerk. He seemed happy with the compromise, but cut Julie's pay back to the billings clerk's salary.

Was it fair that Julie lost a position she'd worked so hard for for years? Maybe not; but in today's competitive workplace, few employers can afford to allow caregivers much leeway. Unfortunately, the burden of balancing caregiving with the workplace falls on the employee's shoulders.

. . . .

Once you've identified and reorganized the work/caregiving overlap, your schedule will be less frantic. By recognizing your own limits as well as your employer's limits, you can balance work and caregiving.

✓

Take a time-management class or borrow time-management books and tapes from the library.

✓

Cut food preparation time by calling the Hearty Mix Company at (908) 382-3010. They will send a catalog of their sugar-free, salt-free or low-calorie prepared food mixes. Or try Avalon Foods Corporation at (718) 322-6000 for a brochure of salt-free cakes, cookies and other foods.

✓

Cut out work-related, nonessential commitments—let someone else plan the company picnic or Christmas party this year.

✓

Take a Saturday afternoon to reorganize your office for increased efficiency.

✓

Pick one caregiving-related chore or task that causes you on-the-job stress, and ask someone else to take over—another relative, friend, community agency or hired professional.

✓

Consider tracking all your own appointments on your caregiving calendar. You'll stay organized and avoid over booking your day. Also, you may be able to schedule your teeth-cleaning for the same day Mom's getting her bridge repaired, or arrange for a lunch with friends while Mom is visiting the physical therapist.

✓

Call the local Area Agency on Aging to ask if they know of any "caregiving fairs" scheduled for your city.

✓

Focus on what you're doing, but don't back away from enjoying your day. If a ridiculous joke or a faxed cartoon makes your lips twitch, indulge in a good laugh; it's therapeutic as well as fun.

✓

Ask employee relations at work if they've seen the "Caregivers In The Work Place" kit published by the AARP. Copies are available, for a small fee, by writing the American Association of Retired Persons, Social Outreach and Support Section, 601 E Street N.W., Washington, DC 20049. The kit contains information on how a company can sponsor a lunch-hour "caregiving fair" for employees and how to develop an elder care benefit package.

✓

Schedule a "caregiving free" weekend this month for yourself.

✓

Send for a copy of "Help for the Working Caregiver" by writing the Health Insurance Association of America, Company Services, 1001 Pennsylvania Avenue N.W., Washington, DC 20004, or call (800) 942-4242.

✓

Post an "is anyone else interested" notice on the employee bulletin board inviting coworkers and management to a caregivers brainstorming session. Do some networking: Does anyone belong to a good support group, know a good geriatric dentist or use an outstanding home health care company? Can you swap tips, rotate errand-running or copy your notebook's non-private resources for a caregiving coworker? Does a coworker have a mother who also enjoys "As the World Turns" and iced coffee? Could you get them together?

✓

Keep stress levels low by taking a one day or weekend seminar in self-hypnosis to relax, or biofeedback to ward off migraines. Check the telephone book or newspapers for adult learning programs. Your local school system may even offer a variety of adult education and recreation classes in the evenings.

CHAPTER FIVE

LONG-DISTANCE CAREGIVING

. . . .

"Dad left a glass saucepan on the stove and went to bed. It exploded and set the kitchen linoleum on fire. Smoke from the melting linoleum got in his lungs.

"I'd just started a new job. I begged my boss to let me off for a few days. I had to pay full price to fly to Baltimore. They said I had to book two weeks ahead for a Super Saver ticket. I said if we knew this was going to happen, I sure would have booked ahead.

"So then I'm driving a rental car in a strange city. Dad's landlord meets me at the door with an eviction notice, because the fire damaged his property. At the hospital Dad's crying because his poodle ran outside and no one can find him. This doctor tells me Dad can't live alone anymore. It was overwhelming. I sat in that smelly hospital lobby and cried."

—*Barbara, motor vehicles clerk, age 53*

LONG-DISTANCE (LD) CAREGIVERS FACE A FEW MORE CHALLENGES than caregivers whose loved ones live nearby. They will likely work harder to get the same results and spend a little more money in the process.

If you are an LD caregiver, to begin, get out your notebook and refer to chapters 3 and 4 in this book. Many of these same ideas will work for you as well. There are some important differences, though. Even when things are going smoothly, virtually all caregiving-related tasks have to be handled via long-distance telephone calls made during regular business hours, which means you're calling during the most expensive billing periods. And while you can gather much of the information needed for the health snapshot by telephone, you know if Dad is looking pale and tired unless someone else notices and calls you.

You can overcome the handicap of not "being there" by looking for creative alternatives, listening carefully and becoming a quality-control monitor.

TELEPHONE TIPS

While you can access the same elder care network as same-state caregivers via long-distance telephone lines, you'll also run up a hefty phone bill. To save on your phone bill, why not:

✓ Ask your long-distance telephone carrier to mail you a chart showing when rates drop so you can take advantage of the cheaper rates. For example, if Dad lives in New York and you live in California, you can call service providers at 7:00 a.m. California time; they'll already be in the office and you will have cashed in on early-morning discounts.

✓ Check out discount long-distance carriers, special bulk-calling deals (like AT&T's "Reach Out America") or preferred-number packages (like MCI's "Friends and Family").

✓ Call service providers, such as medical supply firms, home health care companies or government agencies, when you know their answering service will be taking calls. Leave a brief message, then let them call you back on their dime. (If you need help immediately, this process may take too long.)

✓ If a receptionist or operator asks you to hold, explain that you're calling long-distance and you would prefer to have your call returned.

✓ Have your information, question or complaint ready before picking up the telephone. Be sure you have Dad's insurance policy number, social security number, or the dates he saw the doctor, etc., written in your notebook.

✓ Eliminate costly back-and-forth calls by requesting con-
ference calls. For instance, get on the telephone with Dad's
doctor and home health care supervisor to discuss his
status, rather than making separate long-distance calls.

✓ Ask service providers to check with you regularly so you're
not initiating all the long-distance calls.

✓ Ask Dad's home health care supervisor or social worker to
tape record monthly status reports on a cassette and mail it
to you. You might send new providers a tape detailing
Dad's habits, personal history, likes and dislikes, and any
special procedure you would like them to follow. For instance, if Dad is shy, ask for a male home health aide. Or
you might mention that Dad can only wear cotton pajamas
due to allergies. If he falls asleep listening to classical music
on headphones, let them know.

✓ Save time and money by calling Dad's local telephone
provider and requesting a telephone book for his area. Be
sure to get the book with business (Yellow Pages) and
government (Blue Pages) listings. Or you can have a neighbor order one and mail it to you. Also ask for a "Senior
Services" directory, usually published by an elder-care
community agency.

MAIL OR FAX IT

LD caregivers can't just stop by a government office to drop
off a form during lunch, or meet with a parent's insurance agent
after work. Since the U.S. mail system can take a full week to
get an envelope from one city to another, consider:

✓ asking the service provider to use an overnight or rapid
delivery carrier when time is short; or

✓ faxing information back and forth—including contracts or
service agreements, billing statements, case documentation
and progress reports.

You won't be able to stop off at Dad's every night to make
dinner, of course, or drive him to the doctor every other Mon-

day, or spend lunch hours picking up his prescriptions. Instead, you'll assemble a team of volunteer and/or paid caregivers to take your place.

With persistence and luck, and if the waiting lists aren't too long, Dad will be fed by Meals-on-Wheels, bathed by a "free" home health aide supplied by county social services, visited weekly by friends and neighbors, ferried to doctor appointments by an Ambu-Cab, and taken to church and potluck dinners by his fellow church-goers.

Most likely, though, you'll be paying for many of the caregiving tasks Dad needs. In fact, LD caregivers usually spend more money on professional housekeepers, cooks, companions, home health aides, chore workers and special service providers than their same-state counterparts.

BUILDING THE LD NETWORK

It's usually harder to bargain-shop for the above-noted services when you live far away. So even if Dad is doing well now, it's a good idea to plan ahead:

✓ Contact service providers—medical supply houses, home health care providers, social service agencies—to find out what services are available.

✓ Have applications and information mailed to you.

✓ Compare providers based on service and price so you won't have to start from scratch when an emergency arises.

Entrusting Dad's care to strangers can be frightening. Surprisingly, most elder abuse occurs at the hands of a senior's relatives, but unscrupulous people may worm their way into Dad's wallet while you're not looking, or abuse him mentally, emotionally or physically.

How can you protect Dad when you live 3,000 miles away? Take note of the following tips:

✓ Identify a willing and trustworthy overseer—Dad's pastoral assistant, a long-time neighbor he is close to, or a highly recommended case worker or home health care supervisor. Ask this person to observe other service providers. If you use a professional, be prepared to pay for "case management."

✓ Ask your overseer—and offer to pay her for her time—to be with Dad when strangers must be in his home. The overseer will be an added safety buffer when Dad is talking with a new insurance agent or meeting a live-in housekeeper for the first time.

✓ Advise Dad to refuse any unsolicited services or products offered by telephone solicitors or door-to-door salespeople. There are con artists and thieves who prey on seniors living alone. If a "roofing contractor" stops by and offers to "fix that storm damage" on his roof, tell Dad to refuse, then contact an established local roofing business.

✓ Call the police department and ask if they could have some officers cruise through Dad's neighborhood. Tell them he's a senior citizen living alone.

✓ Hire a private security firm and arrange for guards to patrol Dad's neighborhood. Ask them to check his door and window locks to be sure they're secure. You may want to have an electronic security system installed.

✓ If you have a sorority sister or friend who lives in the same city, ask if they know of a reputable cleaning woman, cook or lawn boy.

When hiring professional service providers, remember to:
✓ Check a company's track record with the local Better Business Bureau or consumer protection unit.

✓ Ask how long a company has been doing business in that location, and ask to talk with satisfied customers, if possible.

✓ Call Dad's doctor, a hospital discharge planner or mental health center in Dad's town and ask for service provider referrals. You also might want to check with the Area Agency on Aging to see if they know of an especially good company for a particular need.

TROUBLESHOOTING

For each LD caregiving dilemma, there is at least a partial solution. Read through the examples below, and then draw up a similar chart in your notebook.

PROBLEM—Dad sounds confused and scared on the telephone, but does not seem to be physically ill. If he can't tell you what's wrong, you might:

- Call a trusted neighbor who knows Dad. Ask her to drop by for a chat, and discreetly check things out around the house at the same time. Ask her to check in the refrigerator to see if he has food and appears to be eating properly. Call the neighbor back at a prearranged time or have her call you collect to report in.
- Call Dad's pastor or a friend. Ask him to check on Dad. Has he noticed a change in Dad's behavior?
- Call Dad's doctor to see if his health status has changed recently. Tell the doctor your concerns. He may suggest hiring an in-home companion or decide to schedule a check-up for Dad.
- Call the Area Agency on Aging in Dad's town and ask for a referral to a geriatric case manager worker who can evaluate Dad at home.
- Ask a relative who lives closer to Dad than you to visit him and evaluate the situation.
- If you find out that nothing serious is wrong, consider paying a professional service to make periodic "hello, how are you calls" to Dad.

PROBLEM—While visiting Dad, you find a stack of unopened bills, an out-of-control checkbook, or piles of medical insurance claim forms that should have been filed months ago. You can:

- Call the local Area Agency on Aging and ask for a referral to a money management company skilled at handling seniors' needs. The AAA representative may also know if any local social service agencies offer accounting assistance to seniors on a sliding scale basis or at no cost.
- Call Dad's bank and speak with a bank representative. Take Dad with you, or bring a note from him authorizing you to get his checkbook straightened out. While there, get the necessary forms to have any income—social security checks, pension monies, dividends—deposited directly into his account (more on this in chapter 6).
- Check the Yellow Pages or with an AAA representative for firms that specialize in handling private insurance, Medicare and Medicaid claims for seniors.
- Ask Dad if he'd like you to handle his financial affairs. If he agrees, you'll need to gather all his financial records, sign various documents and probably consult with an attorney or certified financial planner (more on this in chapter 6).

PROBLEM—Someone calls to say Dad is losing weight, wandering around the neighborhood, wearing the same clothes all week, or leaving his dog outside, unfed. Here's what you can do:

- Call the AAA representative, county mental health center, county health department, or social service department and ask to have a nurse or medical social worker visit Dad at home and then report back to you. If you can't wait, contact the local police and ask them to check on Dad.
- Call Dad's doctor to check on his health and ask for referrals to a reputable home health care provider. If he has been in a hospital or nursing home, call a discharge planner or social

worker at the facility and ask for the same information. If necessary, schedule Dad for a checkup with the doctor and ask a neighbor or friend to drive him to the doctor's office.

- If you know of a reputable home health care provider in Dad's area, ask the provider to send a nurse or medical social worker to assess Dad's health and living environment. Arrange to have a neighbor, fellow church-goer or friend there when the provider's employee visits.
- If an old friend, neighbor or coworker still lives in the same town as Dad, ask him for suggestions on where to get help.

PROBLEM—Dad's doctor calls to say Dad has gotten quite frail and is falling frequently. He suggests hiring a companion, choreworker or home health aide, and adds that it might be a good idea to buy him a walker or put safety rails in the bathroom. You can:

- Call the National Association for Home Care at 1-800-488-3841 and ask for referrals in Dad's area. They maintain lists of home health care companies in each state that belong to this national organization.
- Call the AAA representative and ask what local agencies provide companions, choreworkers or home health care assistants to low-income seniors. Also ask how to arrange for Meals-on-Wheels or medical transportation, names of local firms that install safety equipment, and a medical supply house that rents walkers.
- Interview home health care providers by telephone. Ask to see proof that the provider is bonded and Medicare- or Medicaid-certified. Inquire about the process used to check their employees' background, training and prior work performance. Have information on the provider's billing procedures, rates and a sample contract sent to you. Be sure the provider can be reached twenty-four hours a day and on holidays in case Dad has problems, and that a registered nurse is on call around the clock.

PROBLEM—Lately Dad has been talking about his "young friend" or "new neighbor." He mentions that this person needed a loan or a place to stay, is doing his banking for him, or wants to take him on a trip. Perhaps this person answers the telephone whenever you call. You begin to worry that a stranger is exploiting Dad. In such a case:

- Call the social services department, police or district attorney's office. Explain your concerns and ask for their help. Someone needs to make a home visit right away.
- Ask someone you trust to drop by without calling first to see what's going on.
- Contact the local elder abuse prevention program in Dad's town and ask them for help.
- Arrange to hire professional service providers to take over whatever errands or assistance Dad needs.
- Consider having Dad's locks changed. Notify his bank about your concerns and ask them if anyone has been designated to do his banking; if so, get that resolved immediately.

PROBLEM—Dad is getting worse, and you sense an out-of-town trip may be necessary. If such is the case:

- Check your business calendar and think ahead. If next month is going to be very busy, take time off now and go see Dad.
- Talk with your manager or employee relations representative. Let her know what's going on and that you may need to leave suddenly.
- Train someone else to take over an important project in case you won't be there at the crucial moment.

ANOTHER SOLUTION

There is a shortcut available to many LD caregivers: hiring a private "geriatric case manager." Most geriatric case managers are social workers or nurses who know the ins and outs of the local elder care network. Ask the AAA representative or social services department to recommend a reputable person, and interview them via telephone regarding their experience and credentials.

There are also a few companies that offer nationwide LD caregiving through a network of local affiliates or associates. Here is how such a process works. You contract with the company to provide whatever assistance Dad needs and the company contracts out Dad's care to a geriatric care manager who lives near Dad. A good geriatric care manager will take care of everything, including enrolling Dad in an adult day care program, interviewing home health care assistants or choreworkers, finding the best grocery or prescription-drug delivery service, or renting a wheelchair.

While geriatric case management services are not cheap, they may actually save you and Dad money in the long run. You'll make fewer long-distance telephone calls, for one thing. And if Dad is getting the assistance he needs, he'll be able to live independently for a longer period. And once a skilled care manager takes over, fewer cross-country trips will be necessary to straighten out problems. You'll miss fewer days of work and be able to plan a vacation—and will sleep better, too.

No matter how well you arrange things, it's likely that Dad will have some sort of emergency that requires your presence. The dreaded telephone call comes, and you've got to pack a bag and leave. Being faced with a caregiving crisis is rough when you're sleeping in an unfamiliar bed, away from your own support network of friends and family. LD caregivers must also cope with a host of emergency-related costs, including transportation (gas fill-ups, rental cars, airline or bus fares, taxis) hotels, restaurant meals and possibly lost wages.

PLAN AHEAD

There are several things you can do now to prepare for an emergency trip:

✓ Find out which airlines and bus lines travel nonstop to Dad's town. Write the carrier's telephone numbers in your notebook.

✓ Keep a "caregiving emergency" stash in your checking or savings account, or avoid "maxing out" at least one credit card so that you can charge transportation, hotels and meals during a caregiving emergency.

✓ Have copies of Dad's keys made, especially his door and mailbox keys, and put them on your key ring.

✓ Write down the telephone numbers for Dad's doctor, apartment manager, neighbor and friend in your notebook. You may need a ride from the airport or a security code to get into Dad's apartment. Be sure they all have your work and home telephone numbers, too.

✓ Identify any potential geriatric case managers. Find someone you feel comfortable with *now*.

. . . .

Now that you've custom-crafted a caregiving network for your faraway parent, life will be much easier. With more time available to you and less stress, both you and your parent reap the benefits of your planning.

✓

Cut down on mailing time by having service providers fax information, bills or reports to your office, if possible.

✓

If you can't use the office fax machine, look in the Yellow Pages for local packaging stores or mail services; many will receive faxes on your behalf for a small fee. Write their fax number and telephone number in your notebook.

✓

Do mail order shopping for special products your parent needs. Call Thorndike Press for large-print books at (800) 223-6121; price kitchen and bathroom aids in the Miles Kimball Company catalog by calling (414) 231-3800; and check out adaptive clothing and accessories for aged and disabled people by calling M&M Health Care Company at (800) 221-8929. You also might want to check out the Home Shopping Guide at the back of the book for other mail order shopping possibilities.

✓

Schedule a few days off work and go visit Dad. Using what you've learned in chapter 2, make his home environment safer and more convenient. Use this time to interview a couple of home health care providers, chat with Dad's neighbors and doctor, and select an "overseer."

✓

If you hire a geriatric case manager, ask for weekly reports via telephone, cassette tape or letter. Chart any useful information on your notebook calendar. For instance, you may want to track how Dad's physical therapy is progressing—"walking 15 minutes daily with assistance"—or note that he'll need new underwear and socks by next month, or record his new home health aide's name and telephone number.

✓

Each time you mail a caregiving-related bill, make note of it in your notebook calendar. If a problem comes up you'll know exactly when and to whom you mailed the check.

✓

Call the Aging Services Network at (301) 657-4329 and inquire about hiring a geriatric case manager. Their toll-free number only works in certain areas of the country, so ask them for that number or have them call you back.

✓

Contact the National Association of Geriatric Case Managers for information or referrals to local care managers by writing to 655 N. Alvernon Way, Ste. 108, Tucson, AZ 85711, or call (602) 881-8008.

✓

Send for free information published by Children of Aging Parents. Write to 2761 Trenton Road, Levittown, PA 19056, or call (215) 345-5104. Enclose a self-addressed, stamped envelope. A list of 200 care managers costs $10.

✓

Talk to your travel agent. Ask if airlines or bus lines that travel to Dad's city will waive the advance-booking-for-discount-fares rule for family emergencies. If you've logged enough airline travel to qualify for mileage awards, ask if the airline carrier will let you use it on short notice.

✓

Send for "Miles Away and Still Caring," a guide to long-distance caregiving, by writing to the American Association of Retired Persons, 601 E St. N.W., Washington DC 20049, or call (202) 434-2277.

✓

Switch long-distance telephone carriers if you haven't received the best possible deal. Check out the special rate packages available with a few lunch-hour telephone calls.

✓

Price voice-mail services or answering machines if it's essential that your parent be able to reach you at all times.

CHAPTER SIX

LEGAL AND FINANCIAL ISSUES

· · · · · · · · ·

"When my mother-in-law was 83, she had a devastating stroke and was left paralyzed. My husband's not the oldest of the eight siblings, but they all decided he should get power of attorney and handle Mother's affairs. He spent weeks getting things organized—sorting through files, going to the lawyer's office, the bank, everything.

"At first, two of his sisters took care of Mother, and my husband paid them a salary. Then they got burned out and quit, so he hired a professional live-in caregiver. Now everyone's gossiping, saying that my husband just wanted control of Mother's money. He can't do anything right now. I wish we'd prepared for this, because now everyone's angry with each other."

—*Shirley, scheduling assistant, age 48*

CAREGIVERS SHOULD BE FAMILIAR WITH THEIR PARENT'S financial and legal affairs. If you need to take over the reins— either now or down the road a bit—this knowledge will make things easier.

Get out your notebook and have a talk with Mother. Pick a time when she's feeling rested, and be direct but gentle. Explain that you'd like to get a feel for her financial status and find out where important documents are in case she becomes in-capacitated, even if temporarily.

This is also a good time to find out how well she is managing, and address any problems. Your parent may balk at discussing finances, or perceive your concerns unwelcome interference. Be patient but firm—you need to know what her needs and wishes are. Broach the subject in terms of "help" rather than "taking over." In most cases, though, you probably won't be mentioning anything Mother hasn't already thought of or worried about.

Start by copying this checklist into your notebook:

DOCUMENTS
- Birth certificate
- Marriage certificate
- Divorce decree
- Social security card
- Military records
- Naturalization records
- Tax records
- Living will
- Health care power of attorney
- Health insurance policies
- Medicare card and records
- Medicaid card and records
- Disability insurance policy
- Will
- Life insurance policies
- Funeral insurance policy
- Funeral instructions
- Cemetery plot deed
- Durable power of attorney
- Home deed and title
- Mortgage
- Apartment lease
- Homeowners or apartment insurance policies

- Automobile title
- Automobile insurance policy
- Appraisals/valuation of collections (jewelry, coins, art)

Next to each document or I.D. card, write down where it's kept. If the documentation is scattered, gather it all up and put all the papers somewhere safe, such as in a locked file drawer or safe-deposit box, or have Mom's attorney keep it for you.

Beneath each item, write down the "contact"—who sold Mom the insurance policy, who prepared her living will or taxes, which Medicare office handles her claims. Be sure to include each contact's address and telephone number, along with policy or I.D. numbers, policy value, renewal date, and other pertinent information.

Your completed checklist might read as follows:

LIVING WILL
✓ Prepared by Larry Jones
   Jones Legal Services
   1234 S. River Dr.
   Denver, CO 80206
   (303) 234-5678
Original located in Mother's safe-deposit box at First National Bank, main office, (303) 222-9876. Key in her jewelry box. Copy at Jones's office, second copy at Dr. Gable's office, (303) 987-6543.

MEDICARE CARD AND RECORDS
✓ Medicare regional office
   Blue Cross/Blue Shield
   987 W. Colfax, Ste. 100
   Denver, CO 80213
   (303) 765-1234
   Claim rep: Sue Lindsay, ext. 136

Medicare I.D. #123-45-0011A. Records kept in shoebox in Mother's closet. She carries Medicare card in her wallet.

LIFE INSURANCE POLICIES

✓ Nebraska Life & Trust
9876 Plaza Ave.
Omaha, NE 40329
(Bought through mail)
Local office
(303) 897-9797
Agent: Jim Smith

Term life policy #459043, value $10,000, renewable Jan. 1997. Located in Mother's bottom left desk drawer.

✓ CNA Insurance Co.
4500 Cherry Creek Dr.
Denver, CO 80217
(303) 765-4321
Agent: Jim Smith

Universal life policy #6333-49012, $50,000 death benefit, current value $7,800. Located in Mother's bottom left desk drawer.

JEWELRY

✓ Emerald brooch and earrings
Diamond ring
Pocket watch

Located in safe-deposit box under Julia E. Stecker at First National Bank, 321 S. Market St., Denver, CO 80217, (303) 567-7654. Key in her jewelry box. Appraisals in box too.

Now look over the documents. Is Mother's will up to date? Has she forgotten to renew a term life insurance policy? Is the key to a safe-deposit box missing? If you need to get copies of missing mortgage papers from the mortgage company or ask the lawyer if he knows anything about a living will Mother remembers signing, write it down now.

Next, go over Mother's financial records with her. You'll need to find out where she has checking, savings and investment accounts, as well as safe-deposit boxes. Again, remember to write down each financial institution's name, address and telephone number, as well as the account number, balance (if Mother agrees to share the information) and the full name the account's under. If she's unwilling to divulge financial information with you, ask if she will discuss her affairs with an attorney instead. He can note her wishes and intentions in writing at that time.

Here's what Shirley and her husband discovered about Mother:

First National Bank of Colorado
530 S. Market St.
Denver, CO 80217
(303) 892-4312

Checking acct. #232-6085
Balance $449 on 5/12/93
Savings acct. #737664
Balance $23,554
Safe-deposit box
Under Julia E. Stecker

United Bank of Colorado
17 United Square
Denver, CO 80219
(303) 757-7000
Banker: Felicia Ramirez

Certificates of deposit
Six CDs @ $5,000 each
Varying renewable dates
Safe-deposit box (?)
Under Julia Stecker &
Michael Stecker

Arizona Teachers Credit Union
870 N. 52nd St.
Phoenix, AZ 85019
(602) 840-5500

Savings acct. #192433
Balance $5,831 on 5/12/93
Under Julia E. Stecker

Prudential Bache Securities   Investment acct. #455-136
370 17th St.   Stocks current value
Denver, CO 80202 $14,503 on 5/12/93
(303) 499-9499   Under Julia Stecker
Broker: Tom Lien, ext. 18

In addition to making lists like these, be sure to get a handle on Mother's income and expenses. On one page in your notebook, write down sources and amounts of monthly income. On another page, record what her expenses are. To determine monthly and annual expenses, use tax and medical records, check registers, credit card statements and service receipts.

Now that you have a better understanding of the financial status and legal arrangements, here are some important issues to consider:

DURABLE POWER OF ATTORNEY
A *durable power of attorney (POA)* delegates decision-making authority to another person. For instance, if Mother gave you POA and later suffered a serious stroke—and was no longer able to administer her own affairs—you could sell her property to pay for long-term care. POA can be given to an adult relative or friend, or to a professional, such as an attorney or financial manager, and can be written to address a single issue. Depending on the preference of the person represented by the POA, the scope of the document can be broad or narrow. See an experienced attorney for details, and be sure the word "durable" is included in the document's language. "Durable" stretches the POA's authority to cover periods when Mother is incapacitated.

GUARDIANSHIP & CONSERVATORSHIP
If Mother can no longer make her own decisions, a court can decide if she is incompetent and then appoint someone as guardian. The guardian is empowered to make decisions about Mother's living arrangements, medical care and related mat-

ters. A guardian may be a relative, friend, hired professional or even a court or agency. There are several types of guardianship—voluntary, involuntary, permanent, temporary, limited and total—and all are regulated by state law.

A conservator is a bit different from a guardian. A conservator is responsible for handling Mother's financial affairs. One person—such as yourself—can be both conservator and guardian for Mother, or the different responsibilities can be split.

ADVANCE MEDICAL DIRECTIVES

A *living will* is one type of advance medical directive. Using this legal document Mother can authorize doctors to discontinue artificial life support if she becomes terminally ill. A living will is a limited tool that in most states can only address people who are in a medically terminal condition. In some states, living wills have been challenged in court.

A *durable medical power of attorney* is another type of advance medical directive. A medical POA delegates decision-making authority on medical matters to another person. Medical POA's are more encompassing than living wills because the delegated person—you, for example—can be empowered to deal with all aspects of health care. For instance, what if Mother is incapacitated and one of her doctors suggests an operation that might help her? Unless you have been designated as your mother's health care decision-maker you may have no say in the matter. You might want to seek a second opinion from another doctor, or you might want to go ahead with the surgery; but without the medical POA, your authority may not be legally recognized. Remember that the document must contain specific language ensuring that the medical POA is "durable."

TRUSTS

A *trust* is used to safeguard and manage another person's property and to name beneficiaries. For instance, a *revocable living trust* allows Mother to have control over her affairs while she's healthy, and designates a trustee to take over if she becomes incapacitated. See an experienced estate planning or elder law attorney before making any decisions, though, because some trusts can cause tax problems or may disqualify Mother from receiving Medicaid benefits.

MEDICARE AND MEDICAID
Medicare is the national health insurance plan for eligible people over age 65. It is divided into two sections: Part A which is for hospital costs, and Part B which covers doctor bills and other medical costs.

Part A covers most in-patient hospital costs, along with limited nursing home, hospice and home health care. Part B covers doctors' services, some medical equipment, ambulance trips, emergencies and out-patient costs. Patients must pay deductibles and co-payments, and make up any expenses not covered by Medicare.

Medicaid is the joint federal-state medical plan for poor, disabled or aged people. Needy seniors can have their Medicare deductibles and co-payments paid by Medicaid. Medicaid also covers other medical costs. For instance, Medicaid may pay for nursing home care when Mother's income and assets are within certain limits. Call your local county social services department to see if she meets the age/disability/income/asset criteria.

SUPPLEMENTAL SECURITY INCOME (SSI)
Seniors whose income is below a certain level can get monthly checks through SSI. Mother will have to meet age/disability/income/asset criteria to participate. For an application and information, call Social Security at 1-800-772-1213.

SUPPLEMENTAL MEDICARE INSURANCE (Medigap)
Since Medicare doesn't cover all health care costs and Medicaid only kicks in once you're very poor or disabled, it's a good idea to buy private insurance, called *medigap*, to take up the slack.

Talk with an insurance counselor first, though, to be sure you're not paying more than you need to for a policy that isn't going to save money in the long run. Consider buying only one, good policy.

NURSING HOME INSURANCE

Spending just one year in a nursing home can wipe out Mother's savings. In some instances, nursing home insurance (also known as "long-term care insurance") is a viable option.

If you think Medicare will pay for Mother's nursing home bills, you're wrong. Medicare covers nursing home costs for people who are so ill or disabled that they require skilled nursing care. Many nursing home residents need supervision and assistance, but little actual medical care or they need only intermittent, limited nursing care. Medicare doesn't cover these people most of the time.

Like medigap insurance, nursing home insurance is a good idea—but some policies may cost more than they're worth. Recently, many states have passed laws to regulate insurance abuse, so if Mother has a policy issued before 1990, you may want to review it. Take the policy to an insurance counselor to see if it should be replaced. There's no point paying premiums if the policy has prohibitive waiting periods or excludes everything under the sun.

HOUSING OPTIONS

If Mother is house-rich and cash-poor, you may want to consider a *reverse equity mortgage*. There are a few different types; basically, she's trading the equity she's built in her home for monthly or lump-sum payments. Talk to a banker about your options.

How about a *retirement community*? Mother would have her own apartment and furniture, be around people her own age, and could maintain an independent life-style. Most retirement communities have appealing amenities, such as activity programs, weekly housekeeping, dining rooms, regular bus rides to grocery stores, or on-site beauty parlors.

If Mother can no longer live alone, you may want to investigate local *board and care homes*. B&C homes may be small (a family with an extra room that takes in one or two seniors for a monthly fee) or large (with 10 to 150 residents). At a B&C home, Mother will get "personal care"—help with dressing and bathing, for example, if needed—and meals will be prepared for her. B&C homes are not medical facilities, though, so they're not appropriate for people with serious medical problems or people who need round-the-clock assistance.

If Mom needs more daily care, check into an *assisted living facility*. Mother would still have her own apartment, along with meal service, limited personal care and round-the-clock security and limited medical supervision.

You may be able to find a *life care facility* in your community. Life care facilities are just that—a continuum of housing "steps" that include independent living, assisted living and a nursing home in separate or adjoining buildings. If her health falters, Mother can simply transfer to the next "step" and avoid the stress of moving to a completely new environment.

Here are some more tips to consider:

✓ Find out where Mother's insurance gaps are by comparing Medicare and her private policies. Carefully read any clauses about preexisting condition exclusions, waiting periods, maximum benefits, and the right to renew or convert policies. Check for overlapping coverage—you may want to drop two smaller policies and opt for a more comprehensive plan. But remember that new policies may exclude conditions for which she now receives medical care. Check to see if death benefits can be prepaid as a nursing home benefit.

✓ Check the status of an insurance carrier's status by contacting the state insurance department.

✓ Some families, concerned that their relative will spend a long period in a nursing home, transfer his or her assets to other family members. *Be careful in doing this.* Your relative could be ineligible for Medicaid for up to 30 months after asset transferring, or a transfer could trigger a gift tax. Check with Medicaid or an elder law attorney first.

✓ Arrange to have her social security and supplemental security income checks deposited directly into her bank account by calling Social Security at 1-800-772-1213. You can also arrange to receive her SS and SSI checks as her "representative payee."

✓ Call the same number and ask for a list of local doctors who accept Medicare "assignment." These doctors have agreed to bill only the Medicare-approved cost for each procedure or service, so Mom only pays co-payments and deductibles.

✓ Ask Mother if she'd like to have you designated as her agent in case she becomes incapacitated. The actual document is called the "power of attorney." You, the agent, are known as the "attorney in fact."

✓ If Mother wants you to have access to her safe-deposit box, the two of you should visit the bank to sign the paperwork, Most likely, you'll need to sign a signature card and be given a key to her box. At this time you may want to inventory what she has in the box.

✓ Have a brokerage firm automatically deposit Mother's stock dividends directly into her bank account, or ask the broker to roll this income back into the portfolio. You'll save time, postage and paper-tracking.

. . . .

*Now that you're familiar with your parent's financial and legal
affairs, you're in a much stronger position, one based on knowledge.
Equipped with this information, you'll be better able
to make decisions when problems arise.*

✓

Consolidate all of Mother's money in one bank or financial institution. Be sure that her account balances don't exceed FDIC levels (currently $100,000 per account).

✓

If Mother's account has more than $100,000, the two of you should speak to her banker about opening another account and transferring the excess money into it. That way her balances will be within FDIC limits.

✓

Are you thinking about buying nursing home or medigap insurance, or do you want to know if Mother's current policy is adequate? Write the United Seniors Health Cooperative at 1331 H St. N.W., Washington, DC 20005 for more information or call (202) 393-6222.

✓

Get a list of local attorneys familiar with seniors' legal problems by sending a stamped, self-addressed envelope to the National Academy of Elder Law Attorneys, 655 N. Alvernon, Ste. 108, Tucson, AZ 85711.

✓

Keep blank medical claim forms in your caregiving notebook.

✓

Make copies of Mother's important documents so you'll have them handy.

✓

Write down the name, telephone number, fax number and address of Mother's accountant, attorney, bankers and other important contacts in your caregiving notebook. That way you'll have the information handy when you need it.

✓

Avoid using pre-printed, generic legal forms. They seem safe and inexpensive, but they may not be completely accurate, or may not reflect changes in the law. Encourage Mother to seek the help of an experienced professional for her legal and financial needs.

✓

If Mother is setting up a trust or negotiating other services, be sure she knows whether the planner's fees are based on a percentage of the estate's value, or computed in some other manner. Some states have more restrictive practices than others.

✓

In many states board and care homes are inspected and licensed by the government. If Mother is interested in moving into a board and care home, you'll both want to check the facility's records. Call the state health department as a starting point. If they don't run the inspection/licensing program, they'll know where to direct you.

✓

Have a talk with Mom about her affairs. Ask how she's doing and if she'd like help in any specific areas. This is a good time to discuss the importance of a medical POA.

✓

Send for a free copy of "Organizing Records & Legal Considerations" by contacting Kelly Assisted Living at Dept. GH, P.O. Box 331180, Detroit, MI 48232.

✓

Contact your local Medicare office and ask for a copy of a booklet called "Your Medicare Handbook."

✓

Order a free copy of "Tomorrow's Choices: Preparing for Future Legal, Financial and Health Care Decisions" by writing the American Association of Retired Persons, 601 E St. N.W., Washington, DC 20004, or call (202) 434-2277.

✓

Find an attorney experienced in elder care issues if Mom doesn't already have one. She may want to have her will reviewed if it's more than a few years old, or if her spouse has died since the will was written.

✓

For low-cost pamphlets on advance medical directives, contact Concern For Dying/Society for the Right to Die at 250 W. 57th Street, New York, NY 10107, or call (212) 246-6973.

✓

Laws on advance medical directives (living wills and medical POA's) differ from state to state. Find out what's legal in your sate. If Mother doesn't have an attorney who can answer your questions, you might call the local bar association or medical association.

✓

Remember to respect Mom's decision-making process and feelings while you're assisting her.

CHAPTER SEVEN

HANDS-ON CAREGIVING

· · · · · · · · ·

"When Dad got sick, he weighed 180 pounds and was six feet tall. The only way I could take care of him was to move him in with me. I work eight to ten hours a day, then come home and take care of him. Needless to say, I've made many adjustments. I had to learn the tricks of the trade, one at a time. I sprained my back, he got bedsores. It was really tough getting it together."

—Kim, warehouse clerk, age 39

MOST CAREGIVERS ARE INVOLVED IN HANDS-ON CARE TO SOME degree. You can learn from anyone who cares for an elderly relative—watch them, ask questions and let them watch while you practice. Let's look at some basic caregiving techniques.

BODY MECHANICS

When you're lifting, pushing or pulling Dad, use good "body mechanics" to keep from hurting yourself—or dropping him. Here are a few things to remember about lifting Dad:

✓ Tell him what you're doing each time so he can anticipate the movement and help out.

✓ Balance your weight on both feet, with your back straight and knees bent.

✓ Don't bend forward from the waist and lift with back muscles—you'll injure yourself.

✓ If you have to turn, don't twist your back. Instead, pivot, moving your feet in small steps.

Ready to lift? Get close to Dad. Plant your feet apart so your weight is balanced, push upwards with your leg muscles and support the weight with your arms. Other helpful tips to consider are:

✓ Instead of lifting, try to push, pull or roll Dad.

✓ If two people are moving Dad, get in position, then count out loud—"one, two, three," lifting on the "three."

✓ Adjustable hospital beds are a real boon to caregivers. Ask your doctor if he could prescribe such a bed. Medicare might pick up the tab. Check into renting an adjustable bed, too.

PERSONAL CARE

Encourage Dad to care for himself as much as possible, then offer whatever help he needs. For example, don't comb his hair and brush his teeth if he can do it himself.

Bathing—If he's unsteady, you'll want to buy or rent a shower bench or chair, and install grab bars so Dad can hang on. A detachable shower head with a hose is handy, too, for washing the body and shampooing hair. Assemble your equipment first (towel, wash cloth, soap, shampoo, conditioner) and then test the water to be sure it's warm but not hot. Rinse Dad off; wash him with a mild soap (liquid soap on a washcloth works well); and then rinse again so that all traces of the soap are gone. Have him tip his head forward to wash hair. Use a no-tears shampoo.

You can dry Dad off while he's still sitting, then help him out and finish toweling him down. Again, let him do as much as possible himself. As soon as he's dry, help him put his glasses on. Have his pajamas or clothes ready, and help him dress quickly so he doesn't get chilled.

Put dentures in a cup to soak at night, and then brush and rinse them. If you help Dad brush his teeth, be careful not to brush for long periods without letting him spit, so that he doesn't choke. Comb his hair while it's wet to prevent tangles; if you blow-dry his hair, keep the setting on "low" and don't hold the blow-dryer too close to his scalp.

Clean his ears with a washcloth while Dad's still in the tub. If he has a serious wax buildup, ask his doctor for help. Keep his fingernails and toenails short with an emery board; avoid using nail scissors if possible since it's very easy to cut another person's skin. Some older people develop very thick toe nails that are hard to take care of. If your parent has this problem, schedule regular appointments with a podiatrist for foot care.

Dressing—Have Dad sit or lie down while you're helping him dress. Shop for clothes with his physical problems in mind—buy Velcro-closure sneakers rather than tie sneakers, zippered rather than buttoned clothing. Buy slippers with non-skid bottoms. Many seniors are comfortable wearing sweat suits or other comfortable "action wear" clothing around the house. Be sure Dad always has something on his feet, either socks, slippers or shoes.

Ambulating—Let Dad hold on to you, if possible, instead of grabbing him and pulling him along. Let him put his arm around your waist first, then gently support him by placing your arm around his waist. In this way, he will be less likely to lose his balance. You can also offer your arm for him to lean on or your hand to hold. He may want to use a four-pronged cane or walker for added stability. Encourage him to pick up his feet when walking instead of shuffling.

Browse through a medical supply store or ask to have a catalogue mailed to you. There are some innovative personal care aids on the market, along with many brands of shampoo, lotion and other products that are not available in grocery stores.

WHAT IS "NORMAL"?

When people get older, they tend to experience a few common problems. As a caregiver, you must learn to distinguish between age-related debility and medical problems that call for a doctor visit.

Dad may be farsighted or more sensitive to light. He may have trouble hearing, especially high-pitched sounds and voices. He may move and react slower, and have stiff joints and muscles. If he gets sick or has surgery, he may recover at a slower pace.

While a slight memory loss may not mean anything serious, disorientation or forgetting things you'd expect him to remember may warrant a visit to the doctor. The problem could be simple to fix: he might have low or high blood sugar, a malfunctioning thyroid or not eating or drinking enough. If he seems confused or dizzy, he might be suffering side effects of medication, or you may be observing symptoms of a serious, acute illness. Serious memory loss or confusion are not a normal part of aging and should be evaluated by a doctor.

To be sure he's eating right, ask his doctor for nutritional guidelines for seniors. He may have already prescribed a special diet for Dad—low fat, salt restricted—that you'll need to follow. Be sure you have a copy of the diet, or ask for a referral to a dietitian or nutritionist.

MORE CAREGIVING TIPS
- ✓ Be on the lookout for cuts and scrapes. Many seniors have poor circulation. A small cut or scrape can eventually lead to a serious local or systemic infection that could become life threatening, particularly if the senior is diabetic.
- ✓ It's not hard to change a bed while Dad's in it. Help Dad turn on his side. Pull up the sheet corners on one side of the bed, and roll them toward his body. Now gently turn him back toward the stripped area, and, while keeping one hand on him, slide the sheets from under his body.

✓ Help Dad get comfortable in bed. If he's in bed a lot, encourage him to sleep on his side, lessening the chance of pressure sores. When he's on his side, position a pillow between his knees. If he has edema (swollen feet and legs), elevate them slightly by sliding another pillow under his feet. Gently pull his hips to the side a bit so his weight isn't resting on his shoulder.

✓ Keep the room warm enough so that Dad's feet are bare when he's in bed (it's important to let his skin breathe). Buy pajamas in a breathable fabric, such as cotton. Heavy covers over his feet can cause bed sores on his toes.

✓ Buy rubber sheets, bed protectors and adult diapers if Dad's incontinent. Keep his skin dry as much as possible.

✓ To prevent pressure sores, change diapers immediately, and layer sheets on top of rubber sheets. Wet rubber and wet sheets will cause skin breakdown.

✓ A foam "egg crate" mattress or sheepskin cover, laid over the regular mattress, can help prevent pressure sores.

✓ Several new products are effective in preventing and treating pressure sores. Ask Dad's doctor or pharmacist for product names.

✓ Buy a bedside commode, bedpan or urinal for nighttime and emergency use.

✓ On your next trip to the drugstore, pick up a pack of extra-large toddler diapers and see if they fit Dad. They're usually cheaper and easier to find than adult diapers.

✓ Having trouble buying adult diapers? Call Kimberly-Clark, maker of *Depend*®, disposable adult diapers, at (800) 558-6423. Or call the maker of *MaxiCare*® at (404) 422-3036—they offer "undergarments, contoured briefs and under-pads" that feature a special encapsulating gel. Med-I-Pant Inc. is another option for people with incontinence: Their *Priva*® products are made of natural cotton fabric, with an absorbent inner layer. They're "washable, reusable and environmentally friendly." Call Priva at (800) 361-4964.

✓ If Dad's had a stroke, elevate his weak side or limbs with a pillow. If his arm hangs down, find a safe way to strap it so he doesn't hurt himself (ask the doctor or physical therapist for suggestions).

✓ Buy a gel pack in an athletic supply store or medical supply house. Keep it in the freezer or refrigerator to be used to treat acute bouts of arthritis or inflammation.

✓ If Dad has dementia or Alzheimer's, find safe, easy ways to occupy his hands—folding clean towels and washcloths, for instance. Put up old photos of Dad and his relatives on his bedroom door, in his bedroom to "cue" him that this is his room.

✓ Help Dad change position on the couch or chair to prevent pressure sores. Encourage him to get up and walk every hour or two.

✓ Use lumbar cushions and wedge cushions to keep him comfortably upright in a chair or wheelchair.

✓ If he can't hear the TV or stereo well, try using headphones. Be sure the headphones are lightweight and fit his ears comfortably. Help him tune in his music or a ball game.

✓ If Dad has trouble chewing or swallowing, help him cut his food into small pieces.

✓ If he has problems spilling while drinking from a glass, buy adjustable straws and see if that helps. Sometimes children's lids are helpful.

✓ Buy a baby monitor/intercom so you can hear Dad if he needs help when you're in another room. Be sure to replace batteries as needed.

. . . .

Now that you've learned these basic hands-on techniques, it will be easier to care for your parent. Remember, though, to always consult a doctor whenever your parent's health changes, no matter how insignificant the symptom seems. If the doctor is not responsive to your concerns, you may need to consider switching to a geriatric specialist physician.

✓

Buy a seven-day plastic "pill reminder" cartridge, and count out a week's worth of Dad's medications every Sunday night.

✓

Limit fluids about 3 hours before bedtime, to manage nighttime incontinence.

✓

Ostomy patients can buy supplies at discount prices through the mail by calling and requesting a free catalog from Ostomy Discount of America, (800) 238-7828, or (800) 231-7828 in California.

✓

Buy caregiving-related items in bulk to cut down on emergency trips to the drugstore or medical supplier and to save money.

✓

If Dad has trouble swallowing large pills, ask the doctor or pharmacist which medications can be crushed with a spoon and then taken with a spoonful of applesauce. (Some medications are timed-release formulas and should not be crushed.)

✓

If a pill gets stuck while going down, gently stroke Dad's throat while he relaxes his throat muscles.

✓

Learn from the professionals. Watch the physical therapist help Dad stretch and tone his muscles, observe the home health aide transfer him from wheelchair to bed, listen as the doctor talks with him about his anxiety.

✓

AARP members can buy prescription and over-the-counter drugs, vitamins, cosmetics and personal care products through the mail. Call the AARP Pharmacy Service at (800) 456-2277. (It costs less than $10 to join the AARP.)

✓

Call a medical supply house during lunch and ask to have catalogues and price lists mailed to you. Ask to have information on equipment rental and installation mailed as well.

✓

Send for a free copy of "Medicines & You: A Guide for Older Americans" by writing to the Council on Family Health, 225 Park Avenue South, Suite 1700, New York, NY 10003.

✓

Order "Eating for Your Health" and "Healthy Questions," two free brochures from the American Association of Retired Persons, 601 E Street N.W., Washington, DC 20049, or call (202) 434-2277.

✓

Call Dad's doctor or a local nursing school to ask if they have pamphlets on body mechanics and personal care for caregivers.

✓

Cooking for a diabetic senior? Contact the American Diabetes Association at 1970 Chain Bridge Road, McLean, VA 22109, or call (800) 232-3472. They offer low-cost brochures on diabetes-related nutrition.

✓

Talk with Dad about his daily routine. Find out what caregiving assistance he would like to receive from you or from others. For instance, he may prefer to have someone else bathe him. He may want a male home health aide rather than the woman currently working for him. Or he may want more privacy and less help—so ask him what he wants before you force anything on him.

✓

Order a free catalog of discount priced name brand medical supplies and home health care products by calling Bruce Medical Supply at (800) 225-8445.

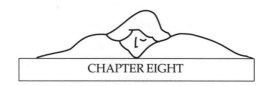

CHAPTER EIGHT

CARING FOR YOU, THE CAREGIVER

· · · · · · · · ·

"My life is a mess. I had a nasty fight with my husband last night because he wanted meat loaf for dinner and I screamed that he could make his own damn meat loaf and to leave me alone.

"I feel like I'll never be the same. I don't have fun anymore, but who has time to even think of fun? I'm sick and tired of doing everything for everyone else. I'm even irritable with poor Mom. Lately she's been calling me by my sister's name, and I said, "What a joke. If Linda were taking care of you, you'd be lying in dirty sheets and eating candy bars for dinner."

"Let me tell you why I'm sleeping over at Mom's these days. Her latest live-in companion took off with her car and the police found it, smashed up, outside a bar across town. The one before that stole her towels, slept all day and smoked cigarettes around Mom's oxygen tank. I feel like a squashed bug."

—Antonia, dental hygienist, age 48

CAREGIVERS CAN ONLY TAKE SO MUCH PHYSICAL, MENTAL, emotional and financial stress before exploding. It's not uncommon to feel:

Grief—because you're losing your mother, the supportive cheerleader you relied on as a child and young adult.

Resentment—because you are always attending to someone else's needs.

Sadness—because Mom has become a stranger with unpredictable needs or frightening mood swings.

Fatigue—because you're holding down a job, running two households, and caring for another person as well as your own nuclear family.

Anxiety—because you realize that no one can keep up this pace forever. Or you know Mom's money is almost gone, or your relationship with your husband is suffering.

Frustration—because Medicare lost her last claim form or your brother insists he "can't take seeing Mom this way" and leaves everything to you.

Anger—because Mom's deterioration is cruel and slow, and other family members aren't helping with her care.

Guilt—because you know Mom can't help being old and sick, or because you no longer have time to help host dinner parties for your husband's business associates, or because you haven't seen your grandchildren for a year.

Fear—because you may lose your job, spouse or financial security, or because you may have to put Mom in a nursing home.

SELF-CARE FOR THE CAREGIVER

Medical research indicates that people who are very stressed—like caregivers—are more likely to get ill. They may develop ulcers, suffer from migraines or catch cold easily. Some doctors believe stress attacks the human immune system, leaving the body vulnerable to serious disease, including cancer.

What can you do to relieve the stress? Experienced caregivers know that they *must* take care of themselves or they'll be unable to function at work, at home or with Mom.

Still, it's hard to fit self-care into a schedule that's already crammed with obligations.

Why not try:

✓ *combining two things that are good for you—exercise and companionship.* While someone else stays with Mom, take a long walk with your husband or a friend, or swim laps with your children at the community pool at least once a week.

✓ *sticking to a regular sleep schedule.* Split caregiving tasks with others or hire out nighttime caregiving to someone else, and get yourself into bed early.

✓ *incorporating a stress-minimizer into your caregiving routine.* Play classical music or soothing "nature tapes" while fixing Mom dinner, sorting laundry or balancing her checkbook.

✓ *caring for yourself while caring for Mom.* Arrange to have your hair cut at the same time she has hers cut. If Mom needs her teeth cleaned, get yours done during the same visit. Take her along to shop for groceries, prescription drugs, sundries and clothing together, if possible.

✓ *visiting the local recreation center or gym to check out the activities offered.* Is there a bridge game for Mom scheduled around the same time as your granddaughter's swim team practice? Does your son's health club offer water aerobics for seniors? Team other family members with Mom—they'll enjoy themselves and you'll get a break.

✓ *finding a support group for caregivers.* Blow off steam during meetings, share your worries and pick up useful tips from professionals and other caregivers.

✓ *reading everything you can about Mom's particular disease or condition.* Ask for pamphlets from doctors, medical social workers and support groups. Check the library for books that explain why Mom's acting like she is, and how to cope with it.

✓ *reaching out to others.* Ask your spouse, children, siblings, and grandchildren to help you and Mom. Don't assume that only you can give Mom what she needs.

✓ *setting attainable goals for yourself.* For instance, when you're at the library getting books for Mom, pick up an interesting novel and spend at least a half hour a day reading.

✓ *journaling.* Spill out the things you're afraid to say out loud in a diary or journal.

✓ *utilizing every single formal or informal caregiving service you can find.* Set limits on how much time and energy you can devote to every aspect of your life, including caregiving.

✓ *talking with your employee relations representative at work.* Ask if the company's employee assistance program has an elder-care referral service.

✓ *sharing your grief and turmoil with someone who will listen*—a good friend, pastoral counselor or professional therapist.

✓ *spending time on simple pleasures.* Bake cookies with your five-year-old grandson, then take him and the cookies to visit Mom. Or send your grandson and his father over to visit Mom, while you take a nap.

✓ *scheduling weekly "caregiving escapes" into your routine.* Some low-cost ideas: a free department store beauty makeover; a lazy morning in bed; a bargain matinee and window shopping with a friend you've missed; browsing the racks in a used book store (bring books to trade in); a picnic at the beach, mountains or park; a potluck dinner and game of cards with your children; a nap; an afternoon at the museum, art gallery, flea market or craft show; a recreation

center class in stress management, self-hypnosis, water
aerobics or stretching.

✓ *allowing time for your personal spiritual practices:* attending
church, meditating, attending a weekly bible study group,
or whatever keeps you fresh.

✓ *being patient with yourself, and keeping a sense of humor as you
go through your day.* You're doing the best you can.

✓ *remembering that nothing, including caregiving, lasts forever.*
Try to keep work hassles and little details in perspective. If
the floor doesn't get mopped, that's okay.

Copy the statement on the following page and carry it with
you in your notebook, or tape it up on a bulletin board or
bathroom mirror so that you'll see it daily.

. . . .
*Taking care of yourself is the best thing you can do for Mom or
Dad. Remember that you have an obligation to yourself:
this is your life, too.*

A Caregiver's Bill of Rights

I HAVE THE RIGHT

- to take care of myself. This is not an act of selfishness. It will give me the capability of taking better care of my relative.
- to seek help from others even though my relative may object. I recognize the limits of my own endurance and strength.
- to maintain facets of my own life that do not include the person I care for, just as I would if he or she were healthy. I know that I do everything that I reasonably can for this person, and I have the right to do some things just for myself.
- to get angry, be depressed and express other difficult feelings occasionally.
- to reject any attempt by my relative (either conscious or unconscious) to manipulate me through guilt, anger or depression.
- to receive consideration, affection, forgiveness and acceptance for what I do from my loved ones for as long as I offer these qualities in return.
- to take pride in what I am accomplishing and to applaud the courage it has sometimes taken to meet the needs of my relative.
- to protect my individuality and my right to make a life for myself that will sustain me in the time when my relative no longer needs my full-time help.
- to expect and demand that as new strides are made in finding resources to aid physically and mentally impaired older persons in our country, similar strides will be made toward aiding and supporting caregivers.
- to (add your own statements of rights to this list. Read this list to yourself every day).

(From: *Caregiving: Helping An Aging Loved One,* by Jo Horne. Washington, DC: AARP Books, 1985, page 299. Reprinted by permission)

✓

Write to the Children of Aging Parents, at 2761 Trenton Road, Levittown, PA, 19056, and ask for a list of caregiver support groups in your area, or call (215) 345-5104.

✓

Do nothing for the next ten minutes. While sitting or lying down, close your eyes and take deep, slow breaths. Relax your body and let your mind float. Do this at least once a day.

✓

Subscribe to "PARENT CARE: Resources to Assist Family Caregivers," a newsletter published by the University of Kansas. Contact them at Parent Care, Gerontology Center, 316 Strong Hall, University of Kansas, Lawrence, KS 66045.

✓

When you see a newspaper ad, a magazine article, or spot a brochure with useful caregiving information, put it in your caregiving notebook for future reference.

✓

Include a "serenity page" in your notebook. If there's a particular poem, quotation or song that helps you cope, write it down. Or maybe you've thought about what this caregiving experience means to you; if it helps, copy that into your notebook. Read over the material for a quick pick-up when you're feeling down.

✓

Let someone else take over. Plan a day off from all caregiving-related duties. If finances allow, hire a professional "respite caregiver" trained to fill in while you take a break.

✓

Call the local mental health center. Find a therapist whose fees are based on the client's ability to pay (called "sliding scale"). Even if you can only afford an hour a month, his or her services could be very helpful. This way, some of your frustration and anxiety can be alleviated.

✓

The next time you're near a bookstore, go on inside. Ignore the weighty self-help books and head right for the humor section. Pick up a Dave Barry paperback, a low-brow joke book or something equally idiotic. Skim the contents and take your smile with you when you leave.

✓

Take yourself to a movie instead of doing something for your parent. In the end you'll both reap the benefits. If you need a good cry, pick something guaranteed to turn on the faucets; otherwise, a comedy is always a good bet.

✓

Call the doctor and ask where you can get literature about Mom's condition.

✓

Call a support group and find out if you can sit in on their next meeting.

✓

Ask any of the following organizations for information on groups meeting in your area:

- Alzheimer's Disease & Related Disorders Association (800) 621-0379
- American Diabetes Foundation (800) 232-3472
- American Paralysis Foundation (800) 225-0292
- American Parkinson Disease Assoc. (800) 232-2732
- Amyotrophic Lateral Sclerosis Assoc. (800) 782-4747
- Arthritis Foundation (800) 283-7800
- Courage Stroke Network (800) 553-6321
- Elder Support Network (800) 634-7654
- Huntington's Disease Society (800) 345-4372
- Lupus Foundation (800) 558-0121

- Myasthenia Gravis Foundation (800) 541-5454
- National Cancer Institute (800) 422-6237
- National Foundation for Ileitis & Colitis, Inc. (800) 343-3637
- National Hospice Organization (703) 234-5900
- National Multiple Sclerosis Society (800) 624-8236
- National Parkinson Foundation (800) 327-4545
- Older Women's League (202) 783-6686
- Simon Foundation (incontinence) (800) 237-4666
- United Scleroderma (800) 722-4673
- Y-Me Breast Cancer Support Program (800) 221-2141

A FINAL WORD . . .

Now that you've reached the end of this guide, you should have your caregiving/work/personal life schedule well organized.

You've learned a whole range of new coping mechanisms. You've become familiar with your parent's health status and linked up with the elder care network. Your parent's living environment is safer and more convenient. You know how to balance work and caregiving, whether your parent lives nearby or far away. You and your parent are aware of the physical, mental and emotional stresses unique to the caregiver-loved one relationship, and are working together as a team. You are prepared to help your parent make legal and financial decisions. And you are committed to taking good care of yourself.

If you haven't already, leaf through the National Organizations and Home Shopping Guide sections that follow. Here you'll find information on where to go for help, where to get free or low-cost advice and where to mail order shop for everything from sheet protectors to telephone amplifiers.

It is hoped that what you've learned in this short book will give you a little more time to do what most caregivers want most of all—to give the aging parent the love, understanding and thoughtful care that he or she needs and deserves.

THE WORKING CAREGIVER SERIES

Caring for Your Aging Parents is part of *The Working Caregiver Series,* published by American Source Books. As the name implies, this series is intended for working caregivers—those who, because of work, caregiving and other obligations, find themselves short on time, short on vital caregiving information and quite possibly stressed out.

If you'd like free information on other titles in this series, write or call: American Source Books, P.O. Box 280353, Lakewood, CO 80228, (303) 980-0580.

Contact the following organizations for more information on elder care topics, as well as suggestions on how to better handle the challenges of caregiving.

Aging Network Services
4400 East-West Hwy., Suite 907
Bethesda, MD 20814
(301) 657-4329
National referral service for geriatric care managers

Al-Anon Family Group Headquarters (alcoholism)
PO Box 862, Midtown Station
New York, NY 10018
(800) 344-2666
Free information & referrals to local support groups

Alzheimer's Disease & Related Disorders Association
70 E. Lake Street, Suite 600
Chicago, IL 60601
(800) 621-0379; in Illinois (800) 572-6037
Free information & referrals to local caregiver support groups

American Association of Homes for the Aging
901 E Street N.W., Suite 500
Washington, DC 20004
(202) 783-2242
Free caregiving brochures

American Association of Retired Persons
601 E Street N.W.
Washington DC 20049
(202) 434-2277
Free/low-cost brochures on home care, elder abuse, home modification, working caregivers, choosing a doctor, caregiver burnout, retirement housing, insurance, nutrition, legal/financial, Medicare, vision & hearing, Alzheimer's, nursing homes (ask for a list of AARP publications); corporate/caregiving education

American Council of the Blind
1155 15th Street N.W., Suite 720
Washington, DC 20005
(800) 424-8666
Free information & referrals to local support groups, consumer-product guidance, referrals to funding sources

American Diabetes Association
1970 Chain Bridge Road
McLean, VA 22109
(800) 232-3472
Low-cost brochures & free referrals to local support groups

American Foundation for the Blind
15 West 16th Street
New York, NY 10011
(800) 232-5463
Free information & referrals to local support groups, sells adaptive-vision products

American Institute for Cancer Research
1759 R Street N.W.
Washington, DC 20009
(800) 843-8114
Free information

American Kidney Fund
6110 Executive Blvd., Suite 1010
Rockville, MD 20852
(800) 638-8299
Free information & referrals to local support groups, financial assistance to needy kidney patients

American Paralysis Association
PO Box 187
Short Hills, NJ 07078
(800) 225-0292
Free information & referrals to local support groups

Amyotrophic Lateral Sclerosis Ass'n. ("Lou Gehrig's disease")
21021 Ventura Boulevard, Suite 321
Woodland Hills, CA 91364
(800) 782-4747
Free information & referrals to local support groups, sells communication equipment

Andrus Gerontology Center
University of Southern California
University Park, MC 0191
Los Angeles, CA 90089
(213) 740-6060
Low-cost brochure on caregiving, elder care counseling

Arthritis Foundation
PO Box 19000
Atlanta GA 30326
(800) 283-7800
Free info & referrals to local support groups, sponsors self-help classes

Blue Cross/Blue Shield of Arizona
Corporate Communications
PO Box 13466
Phoenix, AZ 85002
(602) 864-4100
Free caregiving guide

Children of Aging Parents
1609 Woodborne Road
Woodborne Office Campus, Suite 302-A
Levittown, PA 19057
(215) 345-5104
Free publication list on elder care topics; national referrals to geriatric care managers

Concern for Dying/Society for the Right to Die
250 West 57th Street
New York, NY 10107

Council on Family Health
225 Park Avenue South, Suite 1700
New York, NY 10003
(212) 598-3617

Courage Stroke Network
3915 Golden Valley Road
Golden Valley, MN 55422
(800) 553-6321
Free information

Deafness Research Foundation
9 East 38th Street
New York, NY 10015
(800) 535-3323
Free information

Elder Support Network
3084 Highway 27, Suite 1
PO Box 248
Kendall Park, NJ 08824
(800) 634-7654
Referrals to geriatric care managers

Epilepsy Foundation of America
4351 Garden City Drive
Landover, MD 20785
(800) 332-1000
Free info & referrals to local support groups, database searches, counseling

Family Service America
11700 West Lake Park Drive
Milwaukee, WI 53224
(414) 359-1040
National referral network of private social service agencies

Foundation for Hospice & Home Care
519 C Street N.E.
Washington, DC 20002
(202) 547-6586
Free consumer guides

Health Insurance Association of America
1025 Connecticut Avenue N.W.
Washington, DC 20036
(800) 942-4242
Free brochures on life, health, auto & property insurance

Hearing Aid Helpline
20361 Middlebelt Road
Livonia, MI 48512
(800) 521-5247
Free brochures & referrals to local support groups, product information for hearing aids, free directory of hearing specialists

Hearing Helpline
Better Hearing Institute
PO Box 1840
Washington, DC 20013

(800) 327-9355
Free brochures, list of hearing-impaired organizations, source list for financial assistance

Huntington's Disease Society
140 West 22nd Street, 6th Floor
New York, NY 10011
(800) 345-4372
Free brochures & local support groups, public education

Kelly Assisted Living
Dept. GH
PO Box 331180
Detroit, MI 48232
(800) 541-9818
Free brochures on home care, Alzheimer's disease, home modification, legal issues from national home health care company

Lupus Foundation
4 Research Place, Suite 180
Rockville, MD 20850
(800) 558-0121
Free brochures & referrals to local support groups

Medicare
address varies by zip code
(800) 234-5772
Free general information, counselors available to answer simple questions, eligibility & enrollment information, referrals to local offices

Modern Talking Picture Service
Caption Film Dept.
5000 Park Street North
St. Petersburg, FL 33709
(800) 237-6213
Free loan of captioned films (VCR & 16mm) for hearing-impaired

Myasthenia Gravis Foundation
53 West Jackson Boulevard, Suite 660
Chicago, IL 60604
(800) 541-5454
Free information & referrals to local support groups

National Academy of Elder Law Attorneys
655 North Alvernon, Suite 108
Tucson, AZ 85711
(602) 881-4005
Free information and referrals to local elder law attorneys

National Association of Area Agencies on Aging
1112 16th Street N.W., Suite 100
Washington, DC 20036
(202) 296-8130
Free referrals to local government-funded elder care services

National Association for Home Care
519 C Street N.E.
Washington, DC 20002
(202) 547-7424
Free/low-cost information on hiring a home health care provider

National Association of Private Geriatric Care Managers
655 North Alvernon Way, Suite 108
Tucson, AZ 85711
(602) 881-8008
Low-cost guide to national referrals for geriatric care managers

National Asthma Center
National Jewish Center for Immunology & Respiratory Medicine
1400 Jackson Street
Denver, CO 80206
(800) 222-5864
Free information on asthma & other respiratory problems

National Cancer Institute
Cancer Information Service
PO Box 7021
Colorado Springs, CO 80933
(800) 422-6237
Free publications & referrals to local support groups

National Council on Aging
409 3rd Street S.W.
Washington, DC 20024
(202) 479-1200
Free caregiving pamphlets on elder care and referrals to local service agencies

National Council on Alcoholism
1511 K Street N.W.
Washington, DC
(800) 622-2255
Free information & referrals to local support groups

National Federation of Interfaith Volunteer Caregivers, Inc.
105 Mary's Avenue
PO Box 1939
Kingston, NY 12401
(914) 331-1198
Free/low cost technical assistance to people & congregations who are developing a caregiving ministry

National Foundation for Ileitis & Colitis, Inc.
444 Park Avenue South, 11th Floor
New York, NY 10018
(800) 343-3637
Free brochures & referrals to local support groups

National Head Injury Foundation
1140 Connecticut Avenue N.W.,
Suite 812
Washington, DC 20036
(800) 444-6443
Free brochures & educational materials, referrals to local support groups; listing of rehab programs, database

National Health Information Center
U.S. Department Health & Human Services
PO Box 1133
Washington, DC 20013
(800) 336-4797
Free brochures on senior health & elder care, taped explanations of Medicare & Medicaid

National Hemlock Society
PO Box 11830
Eugene, OR 97440
(503) 342-5748
Free information on euthanasia and referrals to local support groups. Sells books on euthanasia and related topics.

National Hospice Organization
1901 North Moore Street, Suite 901
Arlington, VA 22209
(703) 243-5900
Free information, list of local hospices

National Multiple Sclerosis Society
205 East 42nd Street
New York, NY 10017
(800) 624-8236
Free information & referrals to local support groups

National Organization for Rare Disorders
PO Box 8923
New Fairfield, CT 06812
(800) 447-6673
Free information & referrals to local support groups

National Parkinson Foundation
151 N.W. 9th Avenue
Miami, FL 33136
(800) 327-4545
Free brochures & referrals local support groups

National Rehabilitation Information Center
8455 Colesville Road, Suite 935
Silver Spring, MD 20910
(800) 346-2742
Free/low-cost fact sheets on rehab products, resources and research

National Shared Housing Resource Center
6344 Greene Street
Philadelphia, PA 19144
(800) 677-7472
Free information and local housing referrals

National Stroke Association
300 E. Hampden Avenue, Suite 240
Englewood, CO 80110
(303) 762-9922
Free information and referrals to local support groups, sells books and pamphlets

Older Women's League
730 11th Street N.W., Suite 300
Washington, DC 20001
(202) 783-6686
Free information; some local chapters active in caregiving-related issues

Parkinson's Educational Program
3900 Birch Street, Suite 105
Newport Beach, CA 92660
(800) 344-7872
Free brochures & referrals support groups, sells books & videos on disease & caregiving

Recording for the Blind
20 Roszel Road
Princeton, NJ 08540
(800) 221-4792
Low-cost recordings of books & printed materials for vision-impaired

Self-Help Clearinghouse
St. Claire's Riverside Medical Center
Pocono Road
Denville, NJ 07834
(201) 625-7101
Free information & referrals to various organizations & help lines

Senior Service Corporation
9200 Shelbyville Road, Suite 810
Louisville, KY 40222
(800) 845-6987
Free catalog, sells products and services for seniors

Simon Foundation
PO Box 835
Wilmette, IL 60091.
(800) 237-4666
Free information on incontinence & referrals to local support groups, low-cost monthly newsletter on process & products

Social Security
address varies by zip code
(800) 772-1213 (use this number to arrange direct deposit of Social Security checks, to change your address, to discuss eligibility screening & local appointment setting)
Free general information, counselors available to answer simple questions

Speech & Hearing Information Helpline
10801 Rockville Pike
Rockville, MD 20852
(800) 638-8255
Free information

United Scleroderma Foundation
PO Box 399
Watsonville, CA 95077
(800) 722-4673
Free information & referrals to local support groups
United Seniors Health Cooperative
1331 H Street N.W.
Washington, DC

U.S. Administration on Aging
State & Community Programs
330 Independence Avenue S.W.
Washington, DC 20201
(202) 619-0724
Free brochures on working caregivers & local resources

Visiting Nurse Association of America
3801 East Florida Avenue, Suite 206
Denver, CO 80210
(800) 426-2547
Free referrals to local home health care providers

Y-Me Breast Cancer Support Program
18220 Harwood Avenue
Homewood, IL 60430
(800) 221-2141
Free brochures & referrals to local support groups, mammogram centers, hospitals & doctors; volunteer counselors

If you are having difficulty finding a certain product for your parent, or you would prefer the convenience of buying through the mail, the following businesses should be able to help you out.

CLOTHING

B&B Company, Inc.
P.O. Box 5731
Boise, ID 83705
(208) 343-9696
Free information. Sells custom mastectomy breast forms that fit in regular bras.

Comfortably Yours
2515 East 43rd Street
Chattanooga, TN 37412
(800) 521-0097
Free catalog. Sells clothing, posture braces, reachers & over 5,000 other gadgets and products for seniors.

Miles Kimball Company
41 West 8th Avenue
Oshkosh, WI 54901
(414) 231-3800
Free catalog. Sells clothing, canes, personal care items, accessories for disabled; also sells kitchen & bathroom aids.

M&M Health Care Apparel Co.
1541 60th Street

Brooklyn, NY 121219
(800) 221-8929
Free catalog. Sells clothing and accessories for people with diverse physical problems.

Support Plus
99 West Street
Medfield, MA 02052
(800) 229-2910
Free catalog. Sells hosiery in variety of sizes, supports levels, weights and styles; also sells home health care aids, bath safety products, walking shoes and more.

COMMUNICATION

AT&T National Special Needs Center
2001 Rt. 46, Suite 310
Parsippany, NJ 07054
(800) 233-1222
(800) 233-3232 (TDD)
Free catalog. Sells communication devices for hearing impaired—stationary & portable amplification handsets, pocket talkers, signaling devices & control units, TDD equip-

ment, closed-caption decoders, emergency call systems, electronic artificial larynx equipment, & more.

American Foundation for the Blind, Inc.
15 West 16th Street
New York, NY 10011
(800) 232-5463
Free catalog. Sells products for visually impaired: watches, clocks, calculators, canes, personal & household products.

American Printing House for the Blind, Inc.
P.O. Box 6085
Louisville, KY 40206
(502) 895-2405
Free catalog. Sells products for visually impaired: educational aids, containers, braille writing & embossing equipment, electronic devices, more.

Maxi Aids
P.O. Box 3209
Farmingdale, NY 11735
(800) 522-6294
(714) 846-4799 in New York
Free catalog. Sells products for visually, hearing and physically impaired.

Quest Electronics
510 South Worthington Street
Oconomowoc, WI 53066
(800) 558-9526
Free catalog. Sells electronic devices for hearing impaired—alerts to ringing telephones, door bells, alarm clocks, etc.

Radio Shack/Realistic/Tandy
300 One Tandy Center, Consumer Information
Fort Worth, TX 76102
(817) 390-3011
Free information. Sells variety of electronic equipment & products for disabled.

Science Products
Box 888
Southeastern, PA 19399
(800) 888-7400
Free catalog. Sells sensory aids for visually impaired; builds custom electronics, specializes in voice technology equipment.

Sense Sations
919 Walnut Street
Philadelphia, PA 19107
(800) 875-5456
Free catalog. Sells products for visually impaired: computer products, adaptive recorders, large print, braille and tape cassettes.

Thorndike Large Print
P.O. Box 159
Thorndike, ME 04986
(800) 223-6121
Free catalog. Sells large-print books.

FOOD

Avalon Foods Corporation
2914 Coney Island Avenue
Brooklyn, NY 11235
(718) 332-6000
Free brochure. Sells variety of salt-free cakes, cookies, sugar-free & low-calorie foods

Ener-G Foods
5960 First Avenue South
Seattle, WA 98124
Free information. Sells low-sodium, non-allergenic & law-calorie foods.

Estee Candy Company, Inc.
169 Lackawanna Avenue
Parsippany, NJ 07054
(800) 524-1734
Free catalog. Sells variety of sugar-free cookies & candies.

Hearty Mix Company
1231 Madison Hill Road
Rahway, NJ 07054
(908) 382-3010
Free catalog.

HEALTH CARE

AARP Pharmacy Service
500 Montgomery Street
Alexandria, VA 22314
(800) 456-2277
Free catalog to members. Sells prescription and over-the-counter medicines, dental products, vitamins, cosmetics and personal care items.

Abbey Medical Catalog Sales
2370 Grand Avenue
Long Beach, CA 90815
(800) 421-5125
Free catalog. Sells aids for daily living, physical therapy and rehab equipment—from reachers to wheelchairs and lifts.

American Ostomy Supplies
6013 West Bluemond Road
Milwaukee, WI 53213
(800) 428-3805
Free catalog. Sells ostomy products at discount prices.

Bruce Medical Supply
411 Waverly Oaks Road
Waltham, MA 02154
(800) 225-8446
Free catalog. Sells name-brand medical & health supplies at discount prices; equipment for home

health care, ostomy, diabetes, chronic illness.

Family Medical Pharmacy
839 South Harbor Boulevard
Anaheim, CA 92085
(714) 772-4840
Free catalog. Sells home health care supplies & products; pharmacy.

J.A. Preston Corporation
P.O. Box 89
Jackson, MI 49204
(800) 631-7277
Free catalog. Sells exercise equipment, walkers, crutches, mats, visual and positioning aids, self-held products.

Ostomy Discount of America
600 Penn Center Blvd., Suite 400
Pittsburgh, PA 15235
(800) 238-7828
(800) 231-7828 in California
Free catalog. Sells ostomy supplies at discount prices; pharmacy.

Penny Saver Medical Supply
1851 West 52nd Avenue
Denver, CO 80221
(800) 748-1909
(303) 455-5501 in Colorado
Free information. Sells ostomy, diabetes and other home health care aids & products; pharmacy.

Temco Home Health Care Products Inc.
125 South Street, Box 328
Passaic, NJ 07055
(800) 546-7845
Free catlog. Sells variety of home health care equipment & supplies.

Worldwide Home Health Care Center, Inc.
926 East Tallmadge Avenue
Akron, OH 44310
(800) 223-5938
(800) 621-5938 in Ohio
Free catalog. Sells ostomy and incontinence products & supplies, skin care products, mastectomy breast forms and clothing, & more.

INCONTINENCE PRODUCTS

Kimberly-Clark (*Depends®* adult diapers)
(800) 558-6423

Maxi (undergarments, contoured briefs & underpads)
(404) 422-3036

Med-I-Pant Inc. (*Privia®*, cotton & disposable products)
(800) 361-4964

WHEELCHAIRS AND TRANSPORTERS

Burke, Inc.
P.O. Box 1064
Mission, KS 66222
(800) 225-8446
Free information. Sells rear-wheel-powered scooter.

Dalton Instrument
3121 Gardenbrook Drive
Dallas, TX 75234
(214) 243-0141
Free information. Sells wheelchairs, canes & walkers.

Electric Mobility Corporation
591 Mantua Boulevard
Sewell, NJ 08080
(800) 662-4548
Free booklet. Sells motorized vehicles.

Lark America
W220N507 Springdale Road
Waukesha, WI 53178
(800) 446-4522
Free information.. Sells three-wheel, electric scooters.

Struck Corporation
P.O. Box 307
Cedarburg, WI 53012
(414) 377-3300

Free information. Sells battery-operated scooters.

MISCELLANEOUS

American Foundation for the Blind, Inc.
15 West 16th Street
New York, NY 10011
(800) 232-5463
Free catalog. Sells products for visually impaired; watches, clocks, canes, calculators, personal & household products.

Maddak, Inc.
Pequannock, NJ 07440
(800) 443-4926
Free catalog. Sells aids for daily living; devices & products to assist in recreation, home management, transportation, grooming & hygiene, home health care & rehab.

Self Care Catalog
349 Healdsburg Avenue
Healdsburg, CA 85448
(800) 345-3371
Free catalog. Sells variety of health products & supplies for disabled.

ABOUT THE AUTHOR

Kerri S. Smith is an award-winning investigative journalist specializing in women's issues and elder care. Based in Denver, Colorado, she has written for dozens of magazines and newspapers. Smith earned a journalism degree from the Walter Cronkite School of Journalism at Arizona State University.

ADVISORY PANEL MEMBERS

The following individuals reviewed working and final drafts of this book to assure currency, accuracy and appropriateness for the general reading public.

• • • • • • • • •

Susan C. Aldridge, Ph.D., is the Director of the Denver Regional Council of Governments' Area Agency on Aging. Aldridge is a nationally recognized speaker and has received numerous national awards for her research and program development in aging services.

Susan Fox Buchanan, Esq., is a private-practice attorney experienced in elder care issues. Buchanan graduated from the University of Illinois, earned her law degree at the University of Texas and has studied at Harvard Law School. She is licensed to practice law in five states, and has written numerous articles on elder law issues.

Pamela Erickson, RN, is founder and Executive Director of Professional Respite Care, Inc., Denver, Colorado. PRC provides direct, in-home care to seniors and case management services to determine appropriate long term care options. Recognized as a local and national authority on family and aging issues, Erickson is a member of the National Association of Private Geriatric Care Managers, as well as numerous local organizations.

Virginia Fraser is the long-term care ombudsman for the state of Colorado. She is responsible for monitoring resident rights and care at over 350 long-term care facilities. Fraser holds a master's degree in speech communication from the University of Denver.

Milt Hanson, LCSW, is co-founder and President of the Institute for Creative Aging, Littleton, Colorado. He has been a caseworker and administrator in public and private agencies serving the elderly and their families. Hanson holds a Master of Social Work degree and a Certificate in Gerontology from the University of Denver, and has advanced social work training from Case-Western Reserve University.

Susan Hellman is the founder of the Senior Health Insurance Counseling Program of the Colorado Gerontological Society. She is the author of *Medicare and Medigaps, A Guide to Retirement Health Insurance*. Hellman received her undergraduate degree from Cornell University and a master's degree from Columbia University.

Lewis Kallas is Executive Director of SENIORS! Inc., a Mile High United Way agency serving thousands of older Coloradans. SENIORS! Inc. has established several innovative programs including computer training for seniors reentering the job market and respite caregiver training for volunteers. Kallas earned a master's degree in gerontology from the University of Northern Colorado.

Maria Kallas is a gerontologist working with older adults and their families at St. Luke's Senior Citizen Health Center in Denver. She is also a trainer for the Alzheimer's Association. Kallas has been a long term care ombudsman and previously coordinated the Kinship Program, a statewide organization for family members of nursing home residents. She holds a master's degree from the University of Northern Colorado.

Mary K. Kouri, Ph.D., is a counselor and gerontologist with Human Growth & Development Associates in Denver, Colorado. She helps adults of all ages make successful life transitions and specializes in helping older adults design productive lives. Kouri is the author of *Volunteerism & Older Adults* (1990) and *Keys to Dealing with Loss of a Loved One* (1991).

Crispin Sargent is a principal with C & S Administrators, Inc., a company that provides health claim processing and specializes in health insurance counseling for pre-retirees and seniors. An educator by training, Sargent conducts seminars and contributes articles to regional publications on senior issues and concerns.

Edith Sherman, Ph.D., professor emeritus of sociology, taught for over 30 years at the University of Denver. Before retiring, Sherman was Director of the University of Denver Institute of Gerontology. She is active in community issues and sits on several boards, including the National Council on the Aging, the Western Gerontological Society (American Society on Aging) and the American Association of University Professors.

John Torres is Executive Director of the Colorado Association of Homes and Services for the Aging, an organization representing a number of elder care housing providers. Torres holds a master's degree in public administration from the University of Colorado at Boulder and is co-founder of the Colorado Senior Games.

If you wish to reach any of the above individuals call the publisher at (303) 980-0580.